Praise for

START HERE

"I believe mental health in children is more important than dental health. I'd much rather my child have no problems coping than no cavities. This book shows parents what they can do to help their kids."

Howie Mandel, comedian, actor, and Bell Let's Talk ambassador

"As a parent who watched and supported my child, who experienced bullying and the emotional struggles that came with it, I'm grateful for *Start Here*—a resource for parents to understand mental health concerns and how to recognize them early, with strategies to support mental health within the home."

Katherine Hay, president and CEO of Kids Help Phone

"Having watched several friends navigate various mental health concerns with their children, I know that *Start Here* is such an important resource not only for parents but also anyone who has a close relationship with a child in their lives. By showing us what signs of potential mental illness to watch for—and what we can do to help—this book is a step towards a healthier future for us all."

**Cynthia Loyst, cohost of CTV's *The Social*
and author of *Find Your Pleasure***

"When you're desperate to find support for your child, navigating the mental health landscape can be challenging and overwhelming. *Start Here* is a thoughtful, evidence-based, and highly readable guide to both understanding mental health challenges and finding the strategies and resources to help—a game changer for parents."

Sandra Hanington and Eric Windeler, cofounders of Jack.org

"A front door to understanding the uncertain, bewildering, and sometimes frightening challenges that our children face in terms of mental health. The authors, both seasoned child psychiatrists, provide helpful and hopeful plain-language explanations of common and less common mental disorders and the types of treatment that can make a significant difference, while reminding parents to trust their instincts if they are worried, to focus on understanding and help rather than blame, and to realize that they are not alone."

**David S. Goldbloom, OC, MD, FRCPC, senior medical advisor
at CAMH and bestselling coauthor of *How Can I Help?:
A Week in My Life as a Psychiatrist***

"This concise, welcoming, and approachable book helps all of us develop a better understanding of mental disorders that occur in young people. It should be a must-read for parents and all those who care about our children."

The Honorable Stanley Kutcher, MD, former director of the World Health Organization Collaborating Centre at Dalhousie University

"For any parent who has concerns about the mental health of a child (and, at one time or another, who hasn't?), this is a must-have book. Easy to read and informed by both practical experience and solid research, *Start Here* is written in a clear and respectful way, respectful of the child in crisis and respectful of his or her parents. And best of all, it puts the family at the center, conveying accurately that a suffering child needs strong family support to surmount his or her difficulties and families need to know how to understand what is happening and how to be there to help."

Landon Pearson, OC, former Canadian senator and children's rights advocate

"This book provides direction for parents and caregivers, and instills a sense of hope and optimism that if a child has a mental illness, there is treatment available to help the child and family manage successfully."

Jana Davidson, MD, FRCPC, psychiatrist-in-chief at BC Children's Hospital and head of the Child and Adolescent Psychiatry program at the University of British Columbia

"As a psychologist, I regularly consult with parents who are feeling overwhelmed and concerned about what to do and where to go to properly assess and treat their children's mental health needs. In *Start Here*, Doctors Bryden and Szatmari share their knowledge with empathy and compassion—not only as psychiatrists at one of the world's leading hospitals for children but as parents themselves. I'll be recommending this book to parents."

Sara Dimerman, psychologist and bestselling author

"An excellent and much-needed resource for parents. Written in clear and accessible language with clinical vignettes as the focus, this book provides answers and practical advice to assist parents in recognizing when their child needs help and learning how and where to find it. A must-read for any parent grappling with mental health issues in their children."

Harriet MacMillan, CM, MD, MSc, FRCPC, founding director of the Child Advocacy and Assessment Program at McMaster Children's Hospital

START HERE

A Parent's Guide to Helping Children and Teens
Through Mental Health Challenges

Pier Bryden, MD, and Peter Szatmari, MD

PUBLISHED BY SIMON & SCHUSTER

New York   London   Toronto   Sydney   New Delhi

**SIMON &
SCHUSTER
CANADA**

Simon & Schuster Canada
A Division of Simon & Schuster, Inc.
166 King Street East, Suite 300
Toronto, Ontario M5A 1J3

This Simon & Schuster Canada edition January 2020

SIMON & SCHUSTER CANADA and colophon are trademarks of Simon & Schuster, Inc.

For information about special discounts for bulk purchases, please contact Simon & Schuster Special Sales at 1-800-268-3216 or CustomerService@simonandschuster.ca.

Manufactured in the United States of America

10 9 8 7 6 5 4 3 2 1

Library and Archives Canada Cataloguing in Publication

   Title: Start here : a parent's guide to helping children and teens through mental health challenges / Pier Bryden and Peter Szatmari. Other titles: Parent's guide to helping children and teens through mental health challenges
   Names: Bryden, Pier, author. | Szatmari, Peter, author.
   Description: Simon & Schuster Canada edition.
   Identifiers: Canadiana (print) 20190136529 | Canadiana (ebook) 20190179643 | ISBN 9781508257929 (softcover) | ISBN 9781982144586 (hardcover) | ISBN 9781508257936 (ebook)
   Subjects: LCSH: Child mental health—Popular works. | LCSH: Teenagers—Mental health—Popular works. | LCSH: Child psychiatry—Popular works. | LCSH: Adolescent psychiatry—Popular works.
   Classification: LCC RJ499.34 .B79 2020 | DDC 618.92/89—dc23

ISBN 978-1-9821-4458-6
ISBN 978-1-5082-5792-9 (pbk)
ISBN 978-1-5082-5793-6 (ebook)

To our families, patients, and their families . . .
who have taught us to be better doctors

Contents

START HERE

Introduction

As parents ourselves, we know in every fiber of our beings that becoming a mother or father is a transformative experience, and one that almost always brings with it multiple red-letter days of unprecedented joy. However, we also know in every fiber of our beings that becoming a mother or father is to commit to a life of worry about your child—about his or her health, friends, behavior, and grades—and, of course, about your own parenting. We've been there too. We have five children between us, and, yes, even child psychiatrists question their parenting techniques. The constant stream of worries can be exhausting: How serious is this drop in marks in grade nine? Should I be concerned that she goes to her room as soon as she gets home? Is he hanging out with the right friends? Am I doing the right thing?

While physical ailments such as broken bones and fevers can be frightening in the short term, it's usually quite clear what to do. In contrast, how to handle your child's mental health is often much less clear, and even contradictory. If a child is skipping school, not eating or sleeping well, or isolating themselves from friends and family, some parents are advised to write it off as "just a phase." Others may be concerned that these behaviors indicate a serious issue that requires early treatment to prevent long-term problems. It's not surprising that today's parents feel uncertain if their child is "normal" or if their mental state is something to worry about.

And the truth is that child and adolescent mental illnesses (also known as psychiatric disorders) are common, with somewhere between 10 percent and 20 percent of children and teenagers globally suffering from a mental health disorder. Half of all mental illnesses in adulthood begin by age fourteen, and three-quarters by the midtwenties.[1] Despite the progress we've made as a society to destigmatize mental illness, many children and teens continue to hide their distress from their families and peers because of the shame associated with psychiatric disorders, and parents are left to wonder how they will know if their child is a part of these sobering statistics.

Now more than ever before, parents need help. We suggest you start here. This book is our attempt to address the confusion, helplessness, and isolation that parents too often experience when a child exhibits signs of mental health challenges or illness. We wrote it to provide you with the information and help you need to support your children. After a collective six decades working in children's mental health, we feel uniquely equipped to share the wisdom and practical strategies we have learned from our patients (and their families), colleagues, and scientific research, as well as our own experiences as parents.

If you are concerned about a change in your child's development or behavior, this book will help you ascertain whether he or she is simply "going through a phase" or is in real trouble. (When referencing children, we've alternated the use of male and female pronouns throughout, but we recognize that some children identify as gender neutral and prefer "they/them" and we support this use.) Each chapter focuses on a different mental health issue and opens with a vignette about a parent whose child is in distress, then describes the family's path to understanding what led to the moment of crisis, and how they learned to help their child. As you read, you will accompany these parents and children to meetings with mental health professionals and learn not only about various psychiatric disorders, risk factors, and warning signs, but also what you can do to intervene early to ensure that your child gets the treatment he needs should he develop such a disorder. You will get an inside look into the mental health system, see how a psychiatric diagnosis is reached, what the treatments for different types of psychiatric disorders entail, and what parents of children with mental health challenges can expect for their children's future well-being.

As the title suggests, this book is meant to be a starting point. It would be impossible to provide an exhaustive guide to each and every mental health disorder experienced by children and adolescents, though we have included a detailed list of resources for you at the end of the book so that you can find out more about specific psychiatric illnesses, and, of course, your child's physician or mental health provider is an invaluable resource for any questions we haven't touched on here. Our goal is to help you figure out if your child is struggling with a mental health disorder and provide you with a road map to help her get the treatment she needs.

The most important piece of advice we can give you is this: don't look away. We know that the fear that your child has a mental disorder can be paralyzing. Parents tell us that merely considering the possibility that their child may be undergoing mental challenges evokes self-recrimination, fear of isolation, and the worry that other people—family, friends, neighbors, teachers—won't understand. But if your instinct is telling you that something is not right, trust yourself. There is more harm done by ignoring the signs than by looking deeper.

Some parents have told us that, looking back, they believe they avoided what was in front of them because of an unacknowledged fear that they were somehow responsible for their child's distress. Don't waste your time and energy on misdirected guilt and self-doubt. Focus on your own well-being and nurturing supportive relationships. Doing so will allow you to better sustain your child and family during what is likely to be a challenging time for everybody.

Lastly, whether you are a parent of a child with a diagnosed mental illness or are concerned that your child is at risk, we want to reassure you that *you are not alone*. The road ahead isn't always easy or straightforward, and relief may be a ways off, but help is there for you. There is a lot you can do to help your child back to a place of safety.

We hope this book will empower you to do so.

Anxiety Disorders

A Child in Distress

Ellie can hear her son's cries over the sound of the tap running in the bathroom sink. She tries the door, but it's locked.

"Jack! Let me in," she pleads. "You don't have any germs left on you. You've washed twenty times already."

"I'm not clean!" he yells.

"Trust me, honey, you are. Please unlock the door."

But he doesn't.

At a loss, Ellie takes a deep breath and reaches for the phone to call her ex-husband.

"Just tell him he's being ridiculous," Dan advises. "You can't give in to him."

"Dan, I've tried that already. I can't get him to come out."

She can hear her ex's frustration.

"This is the third night this week you've called me for help with Jack. Maggie and I are in the middle of dinner. I can't manage him all the time."

Ellie blinks back tears. Dan and his new wife, Maggie, seem to handle Jack better than she does. And they're better with her younger son, Ethan, who is nine. Ellie feels pangs of inadequacy when Jack and Ethan tell her about Maggie taking them to a climbing gym or helping with challenging homework. Isn't Ellie supposed to be doing those things? It's been eight years since Ellie and Dan's divorce, and Ellie stills feels a sense of failure, but she knows the divorce isn't what caused Jack's anxiety.

Even as a toddler, Jack had difficulty with new people and places, and he resisted changes to his routine. She remembers him hiding under furniture when the babysitter came. Dan would insist they go out regardless. "Let's go. We're just rewarding this behavior by staying." But Ellie felt pierced by Jack's tear-stained cheeks, dripping nose, and trembling lips.

It was the same when he started kindergarten. Jack would refuse to go. He'd sit in a corner by himself, twirling his hair incessantly while staring out the window. Ethan, on the other hand, seemed to sail through life, engaging strangers with smiles and questions. People are drawn to Ethan, and wary of Jack's reserve and apparent lack of interest.

In first grade, Jack peed himself in school because he was afraid to tell a supply teacher he needed to go to the bathroom. He suffered his classmates' teasing for months afterwards. What followed were years of constipation, stomachaches, and stained underwear because Jack would wait until the end of the day to use the bathroom at home.

Now that Jack is older, his anxiety manifests in different ways. He won't speak up in class, and he rips up all his work if he makes a single mistake. The school principal talked to Ellie and Dan about possible anxiety problems. It was only then that Ellie realized she had never given Jack's struggles a label because she hoped he would grow out of them. But when Jack's grandfather passed away a few months ago, their son took his death hard.

There's a pause on the line, and Ellie can hear Maggie's voice in the background.

"Listen, Ellie," Dan begins, "Jack needs help coping. It's time to get professional help."

They've been through this before, but now Ellie is certain he's right. "I'll call Dr. Khan tomorrow. Please tell Maggie I'm sorry for interrupting your evening."

After she hangs up, Jack emerges from the bathroom. His hands are cracked and bleeding. She opens her arms to give him a hug, and he moves towards her, then pauses.

"Mama, did you wash your hands after you cooked the chicken for dinner?"

Part of her wants to explode, to tell him to just stop being ridiculous, and the other part just wants to hold him.

"I'm going to get into my pajamas," she says, "then let's snuggle and watch some TV together before you go to bed, okay? And let's put some cream on your hands."

Jack nods, and Ellie watches him walk towards his room. What will the pediatrician say about Jack? And how will they all cope with whatever comes next?

What is an anxiety disorder?

We all feel anxious at times, and for most children, anxiety is a normal and necessary experience that helps them develop the skills to manage stress. Jack, for instance, clearly underwent separation anxiety—a child's reluctance to be apart from his or her parents—which is to be expected in children between ages three and four. But as Jack grew up, his anxiety only increased, and Ellie and Dan now realize it is interfering with his ability to achieve important milestones. When anxiety prevents a child from attaining important developmental tasks, such as sleeping alone at an appropriate age, attending school, and participating in social relationships outside the home, and causes them extraordinary distress, it becomes a disorder.

Anxiety is an experience of intense unease, fear, and, often, physical discomfort, usually triggered by exposure to some sort of perceived threat in our environment that alerts our body's arousal response. In other words, it tells us when we're in danger. Anxiety has three components: (1) worried thoughts (a cognitive response), (2) bodily reactions (physiological), and (3) emotional reactions.[1] Sufferers of an anxiety disorder are unable to distinguish between real, immediate dangers and fears that are unrealistic; instead, they respond with full arousal to situations that most people would view as safe.[2] We saw this with Jack's compulsive hand washing despite Ellie's accurate reassurances that he was in no danger of becoming unwell.

If you are concerned about your child developing an anxiety disorder, you are far from alone. There is persuasive scientific evidence suggesting that anxiety disorders are likely the most common mental health issue experienced by children and adolescents.[3] Research shows a worrying rise in rates of childhood emotional problems (which include depression and anxiety) in developed countries, particularly in adolescents.[4] Some commentators have cited the impact of economic uncertainty on families, an increase in academic pressures, and the rise of a consumerist culture as potential causes. But it may also be that parents and children are more educated regarding mental health and so are bringing issues to clinicians more readily than in the past, allowing for more extensive diagnoses. Whatever the reason for the increase, the good news is that we have highly effective treatments for children and teenagers suffering from anxiety disorders.

What are the different types of anxiety disorders and their warning signs?

Anxiety disorders are sometimes invisible to parents—and even health care professionals—because children rarely articulate their anxiety. Instead, they often present with physical symptoms such as stomachaches, headaches, and dizziness, or they refuse to engage in academic, extracurricular, or social activities, complaining they don't feel well. If you notice these warning signs, we recommend having your child's medical symptoms assessed. If your pediatrician or family physician can't find a physiological cause, your child may be suffering from an anxiety disorder. In older children, parents may focus on more obviously concerning behaviors such as drinking and drug use or what appears to be oppositional and defiant behavior, all of which can point to an underlying anxiety disorder. Apart from these symptoms, there are also other, subtle behaviors that suggest different types of anxiety disorders, and it's important to remember that children can have more than one kind of anxiety disorder at a time. Below we've outlined the various disorders in more detail. Again, we cannot emphasize too strongly: if you are observing some of these behaviors in your child, talk to their primary care doctor as soon as possible and ask if your child should be referred to a mental health professional experienced in diagnosing and treating children and adolescents.

Separation Anxiety

As we've discussed above, separation anxiety tends to emerge first among the other anxiety symptoms because it relates to an early developmental milestone: being away from a parent or caregiver. It is entirely expected that a baby or infant may cry when left with strangers for the first time. With practice being apart from parents and increased familiarity with new people, this behavior generally disappears. Some toddlers, however, like Jack, adamantly resist being left alone with even familiar babysitters or relatives and don't settle with soothing and distraction. These children are described as having a separation anxiety disorder. For these kids, starting day care or kindergarten can mean tortured months of crying, tantrums at the entrance, and clinging to parents. Older children can experience separation anxiety, too. For example, a ten-year-old may not be able to cope with sleeping over at a friend's house, an overnight school trip, or summer camp, and if his parents go out for an evening, he may call them multiple times. Separation anxiety can also reemerge in adolescence, manifesting in physical symptoms such as chronic headaches, fatigue, stomachaches, dizziness, and poor school attendance. The longer that anxious children are away from school, the harder it is to help them return. So, if your child is absent from school on a regular basis, he should be seen by a health professional as soon as possible to rule out both a physiological cause for his symptoms and an anxiety disorder.

Social Anxiety

Many children—and adults!—are shy and take a while getting comfortable with new people. With time, shy children will relax and enjoy the company of others. In contrast, socially anxious children find the prospect of others' judgement horrifying and consistently avoid situations where they believe they may experience criticism or embarrassment. A child with social anxiety will generally experience giving a class presentation as nerve-racking, ordering food in a restaurant or approaching a salesperson for help as excruciating, and meeting new people as agony. They may spend hours wondering what to wear the next day to school or rehearsing comments to peers because they are afraid of being mocked.

As children get older, untreated social anxiety may contribute to missed days from school, isolation from other children, and an unhealthy desire to stay as close to home as possible.

Generalized Anxiety Disorder (GAD)

Generalized anxiety disorder describes children who worry about their day-to-day activities and events during many of their waking hours. GAD typically emerges in preschool children, but it can also develop in school-age kids and adolescents. Children with GAD feel physically keyed up and tense. They stress about all the things that could go wrong in their day, in the future, and in the wider world. In some cases, their worries may overlap with separation anxiety and focus on loved ones being in danger. Younger children are sometimes unable to name what they are feeling, but as mentioned, they may complain of frequent stomachaches and headaches that have no physiological cause. Other children become convinced that they have a terrible illness and that every bodily twinge is a harbinger of doom.

Panic Attacks

When adolescents become overwhelmed by their anxiety, they experience panic attacks. They have heart palpitations, shortness of breath, dizziness, light-headedness, numbness, tingling sensations, and an intense fear that something terrible is happening to them. In extreme versions, children can faint or vomit. Over time, specific situations can trigger these panic attacks and, like social anxiety, lead to a fear of leaving the house and avoidance of public spaces and crowds, also known as agoraphobia. While young children can have panic attacks, it's typically in adolescence that they manifest as a panic disorder that interferes with their social and educational milestones.

Post-Traumatic Stress Disorder (PTSD)

While post-traumatic stress disorder isn't considered an anxiety disorder but rather a response to a terrifying life event or experience, we want to mention it here because in recent decades, many parents have expressed their concern about the extent to which children are exposed to traumatic events through the Internet and social media and have wondered what they can do to minimize their child's risk. There is also some overlap between treatments for PTSD and certain anxiety disorders.

PTSD is caused by a child's having direct involvement with, or simply witnessing or learning about, a potentially life-threatening event such as serious car accidents, house fires, terrorist attacks, mass shootings, natural catastrophes, and emotional, physical, or sexual abuse. Children with PTSD will experience nightmares, intense memories (so-called flashbacks, where they feel as though they are reliving the event), and a hypersensitive arousal response characterized by irritability, outbursts, recklessness, disturbed sleep, and problems concentrating. They may also experience memory problems and express negative, exaggerated beliefs about themselves, other people, and the future—for example, saying things such as "What happened was all my fault," "I can never trust anyone," or "I'll never be free of this and achieve anything in my life." Sounds or visual cues or smells that evoke the traumatic event startle them, and they frequently go to extreme lengths to avoid any reminders of the trauma. They may isolate themselves and disengage from activities they enjoyed previously. Younger children may repetitively re-create the traumatic event in their play.

Obsessive-Compulsive Disorder (OCD)

Obsessive-compulsive disorder describes children who experience intrusive and repetitive thoughts—obsessions—that they are unable to get rid of even though they know the thought does not make sense and is causing them great distress. Many, but not all, sufferers try to deal with these thoughts through repetitive ritualized behaviors—compulsions—that initially soothe them: for example, Jack's excessive washing. But when these compulsions inevitably fail to continue to alleviate the distress caused by the obsessions, they become part of a torturous cycle of ever-increasing and desperate repetition.

Like PTSD, OCD has recently been reclassified as its own category of disorder, but we have included it in this chapter because it continues to be referred to and treated by many mental health professionals as an anxiety disorder. What's more, therapy and medications used to treat anxiety disorders can also be effective for treating OCD, with some modifications.

Other Anxiety Disorders

Disorder	Description	Examples
Phobias	While many children have fears, if they are unable to overcome their fear after reaching an age when they would be expected to outgrow it, then their fear may have become a specific phobia.	• needles • the dark • heights • storms • clowns • dogs • snakes • insects

Disorder	Description	Examples
Body-focused repetitive behaviors (BFRBs)	These occur when children with anxiety or OCD, and sometimes other diagnoses, habitually "groom" a part of their body to soothe themselves to an extent that becomes harmful. You may think that most people have these types of habits, but children with these diagnoses exhibit behaviors that cause distress or impairment and that prevent them from enjoying and participating in their day-to-day activities. In severe cases, these behaviors can lead to baldness, a lack of eyelashes and eyebrows, or skin wounds that require medical intervention.	• hair pulling (trichotillomania) • skin picking (excoriation) • nose picking • nail biting • lip biting • cheek biting

What are the risk factors for developing an anxiety disorder?

Risk factors for psychiatric disorders, including anxiety disorders, can be environmental, biological (including genetic), and psychological.

Environmental Factors

Earlier, we mentioned some possible explanations for why anxiety disorders appear to be on the rise among children and young adults. Social media and electronic devices are also a big part of that conversation. Some clinicians believe that alarming news about terrorism, climate change, violence, economic instability, and global unrest—now accessible to children through their phones, tablets, and computers—combined with the adverse impact of those same devices on their sleep and physical activity patterns, have contributed to real increases in childhood anxiety. In the past decade, these devices have disrupted our day-to-day routines by allowing work to intrude into what has historically been family time. Social media has exposed children not just to cyber bullying but also to a mentality of comparison, whether that's between peers or with celebrities.

The last thing we want to do is make parents think that they are the cause of their children's anxiety, but we would be remiss not to mention the popular belief that some parenting styles, colloquially referred to as "helicopter" and "snow-plough" parenting, shield children from danger and disappointment at the expense of developing independent coping skills, something that becomes apparent when the child leaves home for the first time or goes off to college or university. While parenting styles are notoriously difficult to generalize about, given the impact of culture, environment, and one's own parenting experience, we do have concrete evidence that parental attitudes and behaviors can have a direct impact on reducing a child's anxiety.

This is good news, because it means there's a lot you can do to exert a positive influence on your child's mental health. For a study of an on-line family-based intervention targeting parents of children who had an increased risk of developing an anxiety disorder based on their temperament, researchers encouraged the parents to help their children to problem solve by exposing them to whatever made them anxious—thus fostering independence instead of encouraging avoidance. The study found that the children of parents engaged in the program were significantly less anxious than those who were not offered the intervention.[5]

Most parents know this from experience. A nervous child looks to us for validation that a new activity or experience is safe. If we demonstrate confidence in our child's ability to succeed at a pursuit, often our faith ensures his participation. If, on the other hand, we look nervous and encourage our child to "be careful" or let him avoid an experience, we have sent two messages: one, that the new experience is potentially dangerous;

and two, that we don't trust him to manage it safely. Inevitably, we will waver occasionally when our child is distressed and begs to be allowed to stop whatever is causing anxiety, but if, for the most part, we encourage our kids to face their fears, then we are doing our job as parents.

Biological and Psychological Factors

Research suggests that our genetic background plays a part in whether our children will develop an anxiety disorder. How we respond to fear—and our likelihood of having an unhealthy response—runs in families. For example, people with first-degree relatives (a parent, child, or sibling) with OCD have an increased risk of developing the disorder themselves, particularly if their relative developed it as a child.[6] In addition, studies of biological twins show that anxiety disorders run in families because of the shared genetic background rather than some form of learning.[7, 8]

Additional research suggests that anxiety disorders are more common among young children with certain types of temperaments; for example, boys and girls whom mental health professionals describe as "slow to warm up" or behaviorally inhibited. These children are cautious in new environments; hesitant to approach and respond to strangers; rarely initiate social contact on their own, even when they know the person; and frequently reject social overtures from other children. Like children with overt anxiety disorders, children with these behavioral inhibitions have heightened levels of a hormone called cortisol, which is part of our stress response system and plays a significant role in activating and suppressing specific physiological functions that allow us to mount an optimal fight or flight response. When facing new situations, children with behavior inhibition exhibit greater physiological arousal—marked by increased heart rates, dilated pupils, and muscle tension, among other effects.[9] Interestingly, not every child with behavioral inhibition or a "slow to warm up temperament" will develop an anxiety disorder. This points to the complex relationship between genes, temperament, and environment that produces these disorders, and reinforces how parents engage with their child can have a positive impact. We've outlined below what parents can do to prevent risk from becoming reality.

What can parents do to prevent anxiety disorders?

Ellie's and Dan's different approaches towards Jack illustrate what many parents of children with anxiety grapple with. While Ellie wants to comfort Jack when he gets stuck in his compulsions, Dan prefers to draw a hard line. The answer lies somewhere in the middle. We recommend that moms and dads teach children to problem solve and to ask for help when faced with anxiety rather than allowing them to avoid stress. In this way, parents offer empathy and concrete support but also show their children that their anxiety can be overcome. While OCD symptoms may not be completely preventable, given their strong heritability, we know that parents who challenge their child to disengage from compulsive behaviors are more likely to help decrease the frequency and intensity of his or her symptoms.

Below are some strategies that you can employ to minimize the risk of your child's anxiety snowballing into a disorder. Since multiple factors contribute to your child's symptoms, you may implement all these strategies and still have a child with significant residual anxiety—and that is by no means your fault as a parent. Regardless, useful interventions will help you and your child to manage whatever level of anxiety you are both dealing with.

- Convey confidence in your child's ability to overcome her anxiety.
- Encourage her to problem solve and address her fears.
- Teach her that avoiding anxiety-provoking triggers doesn't eliminate the fear of them. Remind her that facing her anxiety head-on is

usually better than experiencing constant fear—and that anticipatory anxiety is always worse than facing the anxious situation itself.

- Talk to your doctor if your child is on a medication that may be contributing to anxiety, such as some asthma puffers and medicines for a condition that we will talk about later in the book, attention deficit/hyperactivity disorder (ADHD).

- Make sure your child gets daily physical activity and a good night's sleep and also avoids caffeine, which can contribute to anxiety.

- Minimize your child's exposure to social media and the news. Separating a child completely from her social group can increase anxiety, so monitor both the quantity and quality of your child's Internet use.

- Ensure that your child has good loving relationships within your family and feels comfortable asking you for help.

- Don't shame your child for feeling anxious; normalize it and emphasize that anxiety shouldn't prevent her from experiencing activities.

- Try not to get emotional when your child resists facing her anxiety. We know this is easier said than done, but if your child is already agitated, the calmer you can be, the better.

If you are concerned about your child's level of anxiety, we encourage you to seek professional help. Early and effective treatment can help minimize some of the negative outcomes associated with persistent childhood anxiety disorders in later life, such as chronic anxiety; depression; substance use disorders; interpersonal, financial, and educational difficulties; and, worst of all, an increased risk of suicide.[10] It is also true that it is never too late to intervene. Below we return to Ellie, Dan, and Jack, and walk you through what is involved in getting a professional assessment for a child who, despite your best efforts, suffers from debilitating anxiety. Then we describe the effective treatments available for your family.

Reaching a Diagnosis

At the appointment with their pediatrician, Ellie, Dan, and Jack are handed simple questionnaires for each of them to fill out and others to give to Jack's teachers. Next, they are referred to Dr. Monique Tremblay, a child and adolescent psychiatrist at their local hospital, for an assessment. After a four-month wait, they meet with Dr. Tremblay and Dr. Azad Singh, a senior psychiatry resident working with her. After introductions, some small talk, and general questions about Jack's symptoms, through which Jack has remained silent or responded, "I don't know," Dr. Tremblay explains that the plan is for Jack to go with Dr. Singh to answer some questions on his own.

Jack looks over at Ellie pleadingly. "I don't want to."

Ellie wants to console him, but before she can respond, Dan says, "Off you go, Jack. We'll be right here."

When Jack doesn't move, Dr. Tremblay says, "Jack, as we've been discussing, your pediatrician has noted that you are struggling with a lot of worries. I know it's hard to do things apart from your parents, but we want to talk to both of you privately to get a better sense of what may be causing you to worry and what may help. After you and Dr. Singh have finished talking, he'll bring you back here to join us."

Jack looks to Ellie. The angry expression on his face cuts her deeply, but he turns and follows Dr. Singh out of the room.

"Tell me," Dr. Tremblay begins. "How long Jack has been struggling with these behaviors?"

"Jack has always had little quirks and challenges, especially at school, but they've gotten a lot worse in the last year." Ellie looks over at Dan as she speaks, hoping he agrees with her description.

"Do you have any idea if anything might have triggered that?"

Dan speaks, his voice measured and calm. "We think it really started when Ellie's dad, Chris, was hospitalized for pneumonia. The underlying issue was lung disease from heavy smoking, but Jack heard a lot about his grandad having an infection that made it hard to breathe, and when Ellie took him to the hospital to see him, Jack had to put on a mask, gloves, and gown just to go into his room. It was after Chris's death that Jack started to obsess about germs. It's so bad now that Ellie can't get him to school on time in the mornings—which, as you can imagine, is pretty disruptive to her work. We've just been lucky her boss is as accommodating as he is."

Ellie appreciates his use of the word *we*. Whatever challenges she and Dan encountered in their marriage, he has always done his best to support her.

"It doesn't sound as though you have the same degree of difficulty getting Jack to school on time, Mr. Fulton." Ellie's face falls, and Dr. Tremblay turns to her. "It's not at all unusual for a child with anxiety to have more symptoms in certain environments than others or to exhibit more distress with one parent than another," she says gently. "And I hope you will forgive me if this sounds like stereotyping, but we often see that children share more of their anxiety with mothers than with fathers."

"I'm glad Jack feels able to talk to me about how scared he is. But I find it incredibly frustrating that I can't get him to do a lot of the things that Dan and Maggie are able to. It makes me feel I must be doing a terrible job."

"You're not, Ms. Johnson. Jack needs you both," Dr. Tremblay says. "An essential part of Jack's treatment will be the two of you working together to provide Jack with empathy and expectation—regardless of whose house he is in. But I am jumping to the finish line. Why don't you tell me about Jack's behavior as a younger child with other children and in new situations?"

Ellie talks about Jack's difficulties starting in kindergarten. He had never gone to day care as she had been home pregnant with Ethan. She did take both boys to activities in the neighborhood, but Jack always wanted to stay close to her rather than join the other children sitting on the mat or playing a game. "Ethan was different, right from the beginning: friendly, outgoing, loved kindergarten from day one. It's hard to believe they're brothers sometimes."

Dr. Tremblay nods and makes a few notes. "Anxiety has high 'heritability.' In other words, it runs in families because of genetic factors. Is there anyone in your family who struggles with anxiety or has been diagnosed with an anxiety disorder?"

"I struggle with anxiety," Dan says.

Ellie is shocked. Her ex-husband has always been cautious, but she would never have said he had an anxiety disorder.

"I was a lot like Jack as a kid," Dan continues. "But having three older brothers, I was forced to get over my fears. I had to eat what they ate, meet all their friends, play sports on their teams. I grew out of my shyness by second or third grade. There's a lot of things that still make me anxious, though."

Dan goes on to describe some of his behaviors: long lists of tasks pinned around the house; a clean, organized workroom; a habit of incessantly counting syllables and steps. As he talks, Ellie thinks back to how many of the arguments in their marriage revolved around her irritation at his extreme attention to detail and his annoyance about her impulsiveness. She realizes now that Ethan is much more like her, and Jack like Dan. No wonder he is able to manage their son's anxiety so much better.

21

"Have you ever had treatment, Mr. Fulton?" Dr. Tremblay asks.

"Yes, my wife, Maggie, made me see a psychiatrist a couple of years after we got married. I started medication and did some therapy, both of which have helped a lot."

Ellie feels a stab of remorse at not being more aware of Dan's struggles when they were married but then reflects that with two children under five, they had both been in survival mode, with not enough energy left over for each other.

She smiles at her ex-husband now. "Thank you for sharing this. It makes me hopeful for Jack."

Next, Dr. Tremblay walks Dan and Ellie through the results of the various questionnaires they, Jack, and his teachers had completed prior to the appointment. Jack's responses suggest that he may have both social anxiety and obsessive-compulsive disorders, which Dr. Tremblay and Dr. Singh will confirm or dismiss in their assessment today. The good news is that Jack did not score highly for depression or attention problems.

"You both noted that he exhibits oppositional behaviors, but his teachers did not," Dr. Tremblay says. "You both described his oppositional behavior manifesting as a compulsion to complete the rituals he believes will calm him."

She tells them that the fact that Jack's teachers don't see this behavior is a good sign, explaining, "It means he has enough self-control outside your homes, which is a sign of strength. It also means he has a good understanding of expectations at school and enough self-esteem that he doesn't want to embarrass himself in front of his classmates and teachers. But he's likely exhausted when he gets home, which is why he lets loose then."

"So you're saying that home is his release valve," Ellie says. "But we need to find other ways to help him relax that don't involve his rituals."

"Exactly." Dr. Tremblay nods. "Once Dr. Singh returns, we'll know more, but I think it's safe to say that Jack is suffering from OCD."

As serious as the diagnosis is, Ellie feels hopeful that they're closer to getting their son the help he needs. "What can we do?"

"A lot. I'm going to refer Jack to our OCD team, which uses a cognitive behavior program that has been adapted for his age group and has proven to be quite effective." She hands each of them a pamphlet. "There is also a parents' group where you can learn strategies to help teach Jack how to resist his compulsions."

"Should Maggie join, too?" Ellie asks.

"It sounds like Maggie has been a big support for Jack," says Dr. Tremblay.

Dan smiles at Ellie. "She'll want to come. She hates seeing Jack in distress. And my brother can look after Ethan during the sessions."

Ellie feels a wave of gratitude. Dr. Tremblay is right. Having Dan and Maggie to help is a huge boost.

"What about medication?" Dan asks. "It's been a life changer for me."

"Good question. Generally, unless the OCD symptoms are severe, we try cognitive therapy on its own first. We can absolutely add a medication if we get a sense the therapy won't be enough on its own, but given that every medication has potential side effects, and Jack is still pretty young, it is entirely reasonable to first see what therapy can do."

Dan nods.

"And remember, as parents, you need to take care of yourself, too. Maintaining your own health is one of the most important things you can do to support your child."[11]

At that moment, Dr. Singh returns with Jack. He passes his notes to Dr. Tremblay.

"How was that, Jack?" Dan asks.

"It was okay. The questions weren't hard."

After Dr. Tremblay flips through Dr. Singh's assessment, she smiles at the family. "It looks like Jack is in good health. His pediatrician already ruled out potential medical causes for his anxiety. There's no need for more blood work." Dr. Tremblay explains that since there is no family history of heart disease, and Jack hasn't reported feeling faint or experiencing his heart racing or skipping beats when he is anxious, he does not require an electrocardiogram.

Jack is relieved. "I hate needles and tests. I'm glad I don't have to do any."

"I am, too." Dr. Tremblay looks at Jack as she continues. "Jack, I've been talking with your parents about you coming back to our clinic to learn how to manage your anxiety—you in a group with other children who struggle with similar issues, and your parents with other parents. Your parents have said they are all in. What about you?"

Jack tenses when the psychiatrist mentions the other children. But then he says, "I can do that. Dr. Singh said that's probably what we would do. He said it will help me."

The small flicker of hope that Ellie felt earlier is growing into a flame.

What are the treatments for anxiety disorders?

As the vignette above shows, treatment for anxiety disorders is multi-faceted, involving therapy and sometimes medication, but it always begins with educating parents and their children about anxiety. Treatment also includes behavioral interventions such as working with children and families to ensure that the child's sleep, nutrition, and level of physical activity support rather than hamper mental health. Dr. Tremblay's recommendation of cognitive behavior therapy for Jack, accompanied by education and support for his parents, is the most commonly recommended treatment for all kinds of childhood anxiety disorders, and the one with the most evidence to support it. It generally forms the core of a treatment plan for anxiety and OCD.[12, 13]

Cognitive Behavior Therapy (CBT)

Cognitive behavior therapy is a type of psychotherapy that helps children look at the links between their thoughts, feelings, and behaviors. A typical CBT session might involve asking the child to identify what makes him anxious—"germs"—and explain why he thinks that. Then the therapist helps the child look at how that specific thought makes him feel—"scared"—and how it affects his behavior: "I wash my hands constantly, which means I'm late for school and slow getting my homework done, which means I get into trouble and feel more anxious." Through education, skill building, and "homework" tasks, CBT helps parents and their child understand what their anxiety is and teaches them coping strategies such as relaxation training and diaphragmatic breathing to manage some of the physical manifestations of anxiety.

For children like Jack who suffer from OCD, CBT treatment would encourage him to face triggers for his anxiety or compulsions through an approach called progressive desensitization, or gradual exposure to his fears. This is obviously a frightening concept at first, so therapists recommend starting small, by (1) simply imagining the trigger, then over time (2) working up to seeing a picture of the trigger, then (3) acting out a pretend scenario, and, finally, (4), undergoing the actual challenge. For example, a child like Jack, who is convinced that he will become contaminated with germs if he doesn't wash his hands every ten or fifteen minutes, will be educated about how the body needs certain types of germs. Then he will be encouraged to touch what he considers "germophobic" items—from a plate to a doorknob to something truly terrifying to him, such as a toilet handle—without washing his hands, all while practicing anxiety reduction strategies. In our experience, we find progressing gradually like this helps both children and their parents build confidence and create realistic plans for managing anxiety during exposure. It also allows them to accept setbacks and frustrations along the way and to keep trying, so that they stay with therapy and don't relapse fully.[14]

The key to effective treatment is ensuring that both children and parents understand the dangers of avoiding the things that make the child anxious: not going to school, not sitting for tests, not taking swimming classes. For a child with OCD, the danger lies in what is called accommodating obsessive-compulsive rituals, where parents allow their children to organize their lives around their rituals, rather than encouraging them to resist their compulsions. This core tenet of CBT for OCD is called "exposure and response prevention," or ERP. While ERP may be used as a component of CBT for other anxiety disorders such as specific phobias, it is an essential part of treatment for OCD, where accommodating a child's rituals only exacerbates the problem.[15] This is especially important for parents like Ellie, who struggle to resist their child's panicked pleas, to understand.

Many treatment programs for childhood anxiety disorders incorporate group therapy so that children can be with and receive support from other kids who struggle with similar issues. And the same goes for parents. In our experience, group programs for parents of children with anxiety disorders encourage collaborative problem solving between parents and provide them with extra support and assurance that they are not alone. Parents have told us that it is often helpful for these groups to have a professional facilitator who can provide factual, accurate information in addition to ensuring that all participants find the emotional support they need.

CBT can be modified for children of different ages, and in some instances, a therapist will work with parents and younger children together; in others, children and parents are seen separately. For older children, figuring out the appropriate amount of parental involvement in therapy can be challenging. Children may have an unrealistic sense of their ability to cope on their own or may resent parental support and see it as pressure.

Negotiating parental involvement with the help of a therapist is essential, as is respecting the confidentiality of the therapist-patient relationship. Years of working with parents and their children have taught us that if your teen doesn't want you to be involved in his treatment, the most successful strategy is usually to offer him independence initially—if safe to do so—with the agreement that if he finds himself unable to overcome the disorder on his own, you will then be invited to participate.

We don't yet have definitive research about exactly how many sessions of CBT therapy are required to support recovery, but the average treatment is twelve sessions. We do know that anxiety disorders tend to have a waxing and waning course, so we recommend that children and their parents think of treatment in episodic terms, and to include booster therapy sessions at times of increased stress. Naturally, there is no guarantee that your child will never again experience anxiety after treatment. But his and your continuing to practice CBT at home significantly reduces the risk of his anxiety impairing his ability to function.[16]

Acceptance and Commitment Therapy (ACT)

Some therapists are exploring the effectiveness of mindfulness therapies for anxiety, including a variant called acceptance and commitment therapy.[17] Mindfulness therapies focus on the child learning to accept his or her present experience rather than becoming anxious about being anxious and to move beyond those challenging circumstances. Studies on the effectiveness of mindfulness and ACT are relatively new, but both are worth considering as supplemental therapy or if your child finds CBT doesn't work for her.

Medications

Despite research that the most effective treatment for generalized anxiety, separation anxiety, and social phobia is a combination of CBT with medication,[18] most patients and their parents opt to try therapy before progressing to medication. For children, particularly older kids, who don't respond to therapy alone, we recommend trying medication sooner rather than later, given what we know about the risks to a child's development and mental health from an untreated or partially treated anxiety disorder.

Because anxiety is a response triggered by our brains, there has been a lot of research into which medications can help manage the body's natural stress response by altering the balance of the brain's chemical messengers that mediate our emotional responses, including our perceptions of and responses to fear. Note that when health care professionals refer to medications, we try to use their generic names to avoid influencing patients to buy brand or trade name drugs that may be more expensive. For example, acetaminophen is the generic name for the pain reliever Tylenol.

-> Serotonin-Selective Reuptake Inhibitors

You've likely heard of selective serotonin reuptake inhibitors, or SSRIs, of which fluoxetine (Prozac) and sertraline (Zoloft) are the most well known as treatments for depression in adults, children, and adolescents. In children and adolescents, SSRIs are actually more effective for treating anxiety.

Serotonin is a natural chemical involved in regulating mood, appetite, memory, and learning, among other physiological functions, and a neurotransmitter, which means that as it is released and absorbed in our bodies, it helps different cells within our central nervous system communicate with one another. SSRIs block this neurotransmitter from being reabsorbed by cells, which in turn leads to more serotonin circulating in the brain, central nervous system, and other parts of the body. SSRIs generally take a few weeks to build up to their full effect, and we tend to keep children who have had a good response to SSRIs on them for at least nine to twelve months after they feel better, as studies have shown that there is a greater chance of relapse when children are taken off them earlier. We also recommend tapering off during the summer months, when children are often less stressed by the academic and social pressures of school.

There are other SSRIs—citalopram (Celexa), escitalopram (Lexapro), and fluvoxamine (Luvox)—but fluoxetine and sertraline have the longest track records and have the most research supporting their use in children and adolescents. No SSRIs have been formally approved by Health Canada for use in children—likely because the available research on SSRI use in children lags behind adult research—but their careful use has been endorsed by both the Canadian Paediatric Society and the Canadian Academy of Child and Adolescent Psychiatry.[19, 20] In the United States, escitalopram, fluoxetine, fluvoxamine, sertraline, and an older medication called clomipramine (Anafranil), which is from a different class of medications known as tricyclic antidepressants, have been approved for pediatric depression or OCD by the US Food and Drug Administration, or FDA.

As Dr. Tremblay mentioned above, SSRIs do have potential side effects, including nausea, headache, diarrhea, either sleepiness or trouble falling asleep, dry mouth, dizziness, blurred vision, and, importantly for some older adolescents, difficulty becoming sexually aroused. While these symptoms tend to improve on their own, children and adolescents appear to be more sensitive than adults to side effects, so make sure you discuss them with your doctor.

More significantly, some children and adolescents are more likely to experience what is called an activation syndrome, where they feel on edge, agitated, and extremely anxious on the medication—some have described this sensation as wanting to jump out of their skin. In some patients under twenty-five, SSRIs have been associated with new thoughts of self-harm and suicide, although there are no reported cases where a suicide attempt has actually occurred as a result of a child or adolescent taking an SSRI. While these unwanted side effects are obviously disturbing to read about, they are no more common or unsettling than the risks associated with a number of over-the-counter or commonly prescribed medications that we take without much thought. Adverse events can be minimized by starting with low doses, increasing them very slowly, and scheduling a doctor's appointment every one to two weeks while the dose is being increased to ensure that your child is tolerating the medication. Having said that, the use of psychiatric medicine is always a risk-versus-benefit discussion. For example, does the potential harm to the child's health and happiness if the disorder goes untreated outweigh the possible risks of using the medication? In general, we don't propose medications as first-line treatments unless by the time we meet a child and her family other educational, behavioral, and psychotherapeutic interventions have been tried with insufficient positive effect or the child's symptoms pose an emergency.

-> Benzodiazepines

The names diazepam (Valium), lorazepam (Ativan), and alprazolam (Xanax) will likely sound familiar. They belong to a class of medication called benzodiazepines, which can provide immediate relief for anxiety disorder symptoms, but we recommend against their use in anxious children and adolescents because they can lead to physical dependence, are likely to interfere with children's cognitive and motor skills that are essential for success in school and sports, and may cause disinhibition and mood swings. Outside of an emergency or surgical setting, there is rarely a reason for them to be used.

After Treatment

It's been ten months since Jack's diagnosis. Ellie leans back in her lounge chair, her hat low on her forehead, watching Jack and Ethan play in the shallows of the warm August lake water.

"You look relaxed," Ellie's friend Sheila says. "Last summer, Jack wouldn't go in the water. Remember? He said it was dirty."

Ellie smiles at Sheila, who has provided so much support over the past few years.

"Jack's been such a star," she reflects. "Honestly, I think I've had a harder time using the CBT strategies than he has. One night a few weeks ago, Jack reminded me that he didn't need me to wash my own hands before touching him anymore. 'Mom, I can confront my fear,' he said. The psychiatrist is pretty sure he doesn't need medication—at least not at this point, given how well he's responding to therapy. We have therapy sessions scheduled until the end of the month, but after that it's on an as-needed basis only. And if the obsessive-compulsive symptoms reoccur, at least now we'll know what to do."

Jack comes out of the water, dripping, and approaches Ellie to grab his towel. He wears a familiar worried expression. "Mama, Ethan says sometimes people pee or even poo in the lake. Do you think that's true?"

"Peeing, yes, but it's not an issue. I doubt anyone poos, but even if they do, it's a big lake, and there's lots of rain up here. There's no need to worry that the lake isn't clean." Ellie looks at him seriously. "Jack, I think OCD is bothering you. Am I right?"

He looks down. "A little."

Before, Ellie would cradle him in her arms and not force him to go back into the lake, but now she knows better.

"Should we tell OCD to be quiet so you can enjoy your holiday?"

Jack pauses, clearly wavering.

"You've got this, Jack. Off you go. And once you've squeezed OCD back into shape, we'll go into town and get ice cream."

Her son smiles at her. "You're right, Mama." He runs back towards the lake, yelling, "Ethan, you're a wuss! No one cares about pee in the lake! Race you to the end of the dock!"

Sheila pats Ellie's hand. "Well done, my friend."

"He's come a long way, hasn't he?" Ellie says.

"You both have."

Substance Use Disorders

A Child in Distress

Hussain swirls his wineglass and looks over at his husband, Saul. "This has been a nice quiet evening in, hasn't it?" he remarks. Their fifteen-year-old son, Marcel, is out with friends, and they have the house to themselves.

"The perfect way to finish a busy week at the hospital." Saul pours a third of a glass, which empties the bottle. "Shall I open another?"

Hussain glances at his watch. "It's late. I probably don't need another. But if you want one?" Saul works hard as an anesthetist and likes to let loose a bit, especially on the weekends. Hussain's job as an accountant, while stressful during tax season, is calmer and more predictable, allowing him to take on the lion's share of day-to-day parenting tasks. Tonight Marcel is staying over at his friend's house, so there's no need for either of them to drive later. "You know what, I'll join you. It *is* Friday."

Just as Saul has pulled the cork, his phone rings. "Yes, this is Dr. Roseman. Yes, I'm Marcel's father." The bottle opener, cork and all, drops from his hand.

Hussain is at Saul's side. "What?"

"Marcel's in the emergency department." Saul answers a few more questions before hanging up. "Someone called an ambulance to the party," Saul explains while grabbing his wallet and keys. "When the EMS got there, he was nonresponsive. They're not sure what he's taken."

"Drugs?" Hussain asks, fear growing inside him. He grabs the keys out of Saul's hands. "Neither of us is in any state to drive."

They pause, shamefaced. "I'll call a cab," Saul says.

The whole way to the hospital, Hussain's mind races with questions. What's going on with his son? He and Saul have suspected that Marcel has experimented with cannabis, but hasn't every teenager? And hadn't Marcel told them that there were parents supervising tonight's party?

When they get to the emergency department, the admitting nurse tells them that Marcel has been taken to the intensive care unit.

Hussain looks at Saul. "That's bad, right?"

Saul nods. "It's not good. But let's not jump to any conclusions."

When they reach Marcel's room, Hussain moves instinctively towards the bed, ignoring the nurse seated at its end, whom Saul stops to question. Marcel's face is crisscrossed by tubes inserted into his nose and mouth and held in place with translucent medical tape. Hussain reaches for his son's hand but stops when he sees the needle catheters connected to IV bags perched high above the bed, dispensing fluids and essential electrolytes.

"Saul," Hussain says, and his husband turns from the ICU nurse.

"He's going to be okay," Saul says, his voice clipped and composed. "They're not certain what he took, but his vital signs are holding. They think he may have taken a central nervous system depressant that has affected his breathing. They're going to watch him in the ICU for the next twenty-four hours and then see if they can wean him off the respirator."

Hussain feels winded, as though he's been punched in the gut. He can barely breathe, barely take it in. "How could this have happened?"

Saul's doctor persona remains intact. "Right now we need to focus on the fact that he's young and strong and likely to pull through. I'm going to stay here with him overnight. Why don't you go home and get some sleep?"

Hussain wants to protest, but he knows Saul's plan makes sense. Still, he wishes his husband would respond less like a doctor and more like a father. He leans over the tubes to kiss Marcel's tousled hair. "I love you, Marcello superstello," he murmurs, then stands by Saul for a moment, hoping for a touch—some kind of reassurance—but it never comes. Hussain leaves.

At home, he wanders into their son's room. It's a mess. Dirty clothes cover the floor, an open hockey bag gives off a musty smell. The only patch of order is the mantelpiece, where Marcel's soccer and hockey trophies gleam.

Sadly, there won't be a team photo this year. During Marcel's first year of high school, his interest in sports seemed to wane. He made new friends who were more interested in parties and girls than in athletics, and he gave up soccer and hockey entirely. He said it was to make time to do better in school, but his marks dropped last year. Saul and Hussain have acknowledged to each other that Marcel has likely experimented with both alcohol and cannabis but now Hussain wonders if there is something more going on. Lately, their son has become withdrawn. Marcel had always been friendly and warm, but he doesn't show much affection for them at all and seems detached. In addition, the teenager's eating and sleeping habits have changed. His appetite has become erratic, and he often refuses to wake up in time to eat breakfast before heading off to school. As Hussain thinks back on all these changes in Marcel, he realizes that he and Saul have been avoiding a tough conversation with their son about drugs and alcohol—and about the example they're setting with their own substance use.[1] Hussain closes his eyes, his head on Marcel's pillow, but he can't sleep. All he sees is his son surrounded by tubes on the narrow ICU bed.

What is a substance use disorder and its warning signs?

In the above vignette, Hussain and Saul are realizing that their son's relationship with alcohol and drug use has grown beyond normal teenage experimentation and has become psychologically and medically damaging. In other words, Marcel is showing signs of a potential substance use disorder. A person is said to suffer from a substance use disorder when his alcohol or drug use causes significant impairment or distress, including at least two of the following aspects:[2]

- escalating drug use despite a persistent desire to cut down or control it;
- increasing time spent on activities necessary to obtain, use, or recover from the drug cravings;
- repeated drug use that results in failure to fulfill school, home, and/or work obligations;
- continued drug use in the face of recurring social or interpersonal problems caused by the drug's effects;
- giving up important social, occupational, or recreational activities because of drug use;
- ongoing use in physically hazardous situations, such as driving or operating potentially dangerous work tools;
- drug use despite the knowledge that it has contributed to a persistent physical or psychological problem;
- tolerance to the drug, characterized by a need for increased amounts to get the desired effect; and
- a withdrawal syndrome if the drug is not taken.

When someone exhibits more than two of the above symptoms in a twelve-month period, his substance use disorder has progressed past mild to moderate or even severe. At one time, we would have referred to this kind of behavior as addiction, but given the range and different types of harmful relationships individuals develop with substances (and the stigma associated with the word *addiction*), we are moving away from the term in the mental health profession. Despite the gravity of this diagnosis, there is encouraging news: you can take specific actions to minimize your child's risk, and, if your child is already at the point of exhibiting warning signs, we'll tell you what you can do to access appropriate treatment.

As Hussain and Saul's story illustrates, one of the greatest challenges for parents of teens is discerning when experimentation is "normal" and when a child is in trouble. Let's look at what the norms are for adolescents when it comes to alcohol and drug use.

A Snapshot of Alcohol and Drug Use in Grades 7–12 in Canada in 2017[3]

SUBSTANCE	Percentage
Alcohol	42.5%
High-caffeine energy drinks	34.1%
Cannabis	19%
Binge-drinking	16.9%
Nonmedical use of a prescription drug*	13.7%
Electronic cigarettes	10.7%
Opioid pain relievers (nonmedical use)	10.6%
Over-the-counter cough/cold medication	9.2%
Tobacco cigarettes	7%
Waterpipes (hookahs)	6.2%
Smokeless (chewing) tobacco	5.4%
Mushrooms or mescaline*	4%
Inhalants (glue or solvents)	3.4%
Ecstasy (MDMA)*	3.4%
Cocaine*	3.1%
Tranquilizers/sedatives (nonmedical use)*	2.7%
ADHD drugs (nonmedical use)	2.3%
Synthetic cannabis (Spice, K2)	1.5%
LSD*	1.5%
Fentanyl*	0.9%
Jimson Weed*	0.8%
Methamphetamine*	0.6%
Cocaine*	0.6%

*Stats measured in Grades 9–12

A Snapshot of Alcohol and Drug Use in Grades 9–12 in the U.S. in 2017 [4, 5]

SUBSTANCE	Percentage
Alcohol	29.8%
Cannabis	19.8%
Nonmedical use of a prescription drug	14%
Binge-drinking	13.5%
Electronic cigarettes	13%
Tobacco cigarettes	9%
Synthetic cannabis (Spice, K2)	6.9%
Hallucinogenic drugs (LSD, mushrooms or mescaline)	6.6%
Inhalants (glue or solvents)	6.2%
Smokeless (chewing) tobacco	5%
Cocaine	4.8%
Ecstasy (MDMA)	4%
Methamphetamine	2.5%
Heroin	1.7%

As you can see above, alcohol remains the most commonly used substance, although its use has dropped from past years, along with nicotine and cannabis. Use of opioid drugs (a class of medications usually used to treat pain, which includes oxycodone, hydrocodone, heroin, fentanyl, morphine, and codeine) has also declined among Canadian teenagers, as has heroin among US teens. Use of other opioids has only recently been measured in US youth, from 2017 on, so it is difficult to speak to a trend yet. That said, while overall the news is good, today's cannabis is much more potent than that of the early 1990s, which means the risks are greater for our kids than they were for prior generations.

Another concerning trend has been a substantial increase in the past few years in vaping, the inhalation through an electronic cigarette of water vapor containing heated nicotine, flavors, and other chemicals. While the majority of teens who vape report that they are using flavored products that don't contain nicotine, this is likely inaccurate because manufacturers don't have to report e-cigarette ingredients. About 6 percent of teens report using products that contain cannabis. These facts are obviously cause for concern, especially given the recent reports of severe respiratory illnesses and deaths linked to vaping. Additionally, about a third of e-cigarette users start smoking cigarettes within six months of their first experience with vaping, as opposed to only 8 percent of people who do not vape, which suggests that e-cigarettes may be a gateway to smoking.[6]

Aside from vaping, the only other recent increase in substance use among teens is the recreational use of over-the-counter cough and cold medications containing dextromethorphan (Benylin DM, Robitussin), chlorpheniramine (Chlor-Trimeton, Chlor-Tripolon), pseudoephedrine (Sudafed); antiemetic dimenhydrinate (Gravol); and the antihistamine and antiallergen diphenhydramine (Benadryl). All of these can cause intoxication and, at high doses, even psychosis—a neuropsychiatric syndrome with multiple possible causes—which we discuss in a later chapter. Despite being available without a prescription, they have considerable medical risks, some life threatening, if used in excess.[7]

As parents, it's easy for us to see those statistics and think, "But that's not my child." And it may not be. Not all children who experiment with substances in high school go on to have a substance use disorder. However, in our experience, teens are experts at hiding the truth from adults—especially from their parents and guardians. Adolescence is a time of exploration and experimentation, but it's also a time when teens are at the most risk for misusing drugs. Young children are also vulnerable, particularly to using inhalants (household cleaners, glue, gasoline, and permanent markers), presumably because of their relative availability, and there are significant medical hazards from sniffing these substances.

Most mothers and fathers are familiar with the dangers of children experimenting with and potentially misusing nicotine, cannabis, and alcohol, but parents may not be as aware of other substances that teens are experimenting with, including stimulant medications used to treat ADHD (methylphenidate and dextroamphetamine, sold under the trade names Ritalin and Dexedrine, respectively) and nonprescription stimulant and hallucinogenic drugs such as Ecstasy (MDMA), metham-phetamine, lysergic acid diethylamide (LSD), phencyclidine (PCP), and cocaine. Other prescription medications that have become frighteningly accessible to adolescents are benzodiazepines (of which diazepam, or Va-lium, is the best known), most commonly alprazolam (Xanax),[8] and the aforementioned opioid painkillers hydrocodone (Vicodin) and oxyco-done (Percocet, OxyContin). There are also the so-called date rape drugs: benzodiazepine flunitrazepam (Rohypnol), gamma hydroxybutyric acid (GHB), and ketamine. New synthetic cannabis variants (K2 and Spice) are increasingly available, as is a human synthetic cathinone (a so-called cousin to amphetamine drugs) called bath salts. This cathinone is similar to but significantly more dangerous than the cathinone ingredient found in khat, a natural herbal stimulant harvested and widely used in East Africa and the Arabian Peninsula, and which, like bath salts, has become more widely available in Europe and North America in recent decades.

We list these drugs not to scare you but to ensure that you have all the information you need to be on the lookout for signs that your child is struggling. It's easy to get caught up in a discussion that one substance is "better" or "less risky" than another. But remember that when used regularly, all substances can leave teens on the precipice of dependency. A recent Canadian study found that 27 percent to 50 percent of adoles-cents who died by suicide met the diagnostic criteria for a substance use disorder.[9] And, of course, there are risks and consequences even from onetime use, such as overdosing on an opioid or road accidents due to impaired driving.

Before we discuss warning signs to watch out for, let's talk about the specific risks of cannabis use, given recent societal shifts in its legality and availability. Six studies from five countries that have tracked adolescents into young adulthood have demonstrated an undeniable link between regular early cannabis use and an increased likelihood of later psychosis and schizophrenia.[10] It remains a matter for debate as to whether preexisting symptoms of psychosis encourage some adolescents to seek out and use cannabis more heavily or whether their use is related to the development of psychosis. Regular cannabis use in adolescence has also been associated with increased risks for depression and suicidality in users when they reach early adulthood.[11]

When it comes to warning signs for all types of substance use disorders, first off, don't be fooled by age. There is clear evidence that some children get involved with drugs as early as age twelve. The earliest warning signs involve changes in your child's behavior and habits, such as:

- a new set of friends whom you don't know;
- withdrawal from family activities in which they previously participated and enjoyed;
- drastic increase or decrease in appetite;
- changes in sleep habits;
- a drop in academic performance;
- school truancy and long absences from home with repeated violations of agreed-upon curfews;
- new angry and violent behavior in response to previous nonissues;
- lack of self-restraint in a child who was usually well behaved;
- increased and incoherent talkativeness;
- complaints of fatigue and other medical issues;
- staying awake at night and sleeping much of the day;
- bloodshot eyes, unusually small or large pupil size;
- chronic cough;
- drug paraphernalia such as rolling papers, bongs, pipes, syringes, plastic baggies, roach clips, and so on.

When it comes to chronic drug use, you may notice other signs, such as a lack of motivation; neglecting personal hygiene and grooming;

dramatic changes in appearance, such as weight gain or loss, new tattoos, and clothes and jewelry with symbols indicating drug use; and antisocial behaviors such as stealing, increased mood swings, depression, apathy, and suicidal thoughts, actions, and statements. Lying becomes inevitable as the child tries to hide evidence of his substance use from his parents. Prolonged use may cause skin and nasal sores, particularly scabs on the arms and legs from injecting drugs. You may come across some of the drug paraphernalia listed above. If your child is going through withdrawal, she may be dramatic, erratic, emotional, and irritable.[12]

While we recognize that this catalogue of warning signs is frightening, we recommend that parents confront this type of evidence and intervene immediately. Children often insist that there is no problem, but we know from our clinical work that, deep down, kids know when they are in trouble and recognize the validity of their parents' concerns and intervention. We have spoken to many parents whose children told them years later that their parents' insistence on treatment saved their lives, even though at the time they responded angrily, even violently.

What are the risk factors for developing a substance use disorder?

Environmental Factors

It won't shock many parents that a child whose friends drink or smoke or use drugs is more likely to engage in these behaviors than if their friends are kids who stay away from substances.[13] Peer influences become stronger with age[14, 15] and the Internet facilitates the availability of drugs, courtesy of a proliferation of illegitimate pharmacies that provide medications without prescriptions or physician visits.[16] Adolescents who are lesbian, gay, bisexual, transgender, queer, and two-spirited (LGBTQ2S) and children with a history of suffering from physical and/or sexual abuse are more at risk of developing a substance use disorder.[17, 18] Despite some societal progress, LGBTQ2S teens continue to experience minority stress—the experience of living in a social environment dominated by the values and mores of the majority, and exposure to discrimination, rejection, and stigma—which may explain their increased susceptibility. We do know that childhood experiences of trauma are associated with a host of later mental health concerns. In our clinical experience, these children struggle with trust and attachment—for good reason—and are fearful when it comes to seeking out and engaging in sustained treatment.

It is good to know that as parents, we can influence our children's environments and structure our families' lives, relationships, and activities, all of which play important parts in mitigating risk. Parents often tell us they don't want to lie to their children about their own adolescent experiences. Honesty is always the best policy, but be aware of how much to say. An eleven-year-old doesn't need to hear about a parent's past opioid abuse or experiences of alcohol poisoning, but a mature seventeen-year-old who expresses curiosity and is navigating her own exposure to both alcohol and drugs may be ready to hear this type of story. Most children will accept a version of the following answer from you: "Neither of us was perfectly behaved in our teens. We both made mistakes which we will be happy to share with you, but the details need to wait until you are older. Right now we need to focus on your choices and helping you to make safe ones, not perfect ones."

Like many parents, Hussain feels uncomfortable thinking that his own substance use could have influenced his child. Study after study tells us that in this area, modeling the proper behavior is the most valuable thing moms and dads can do. If a parent has his own alcohol and substance use issues, not only is he modeling unsafe behavior, but also he is less able to provide adequate parental monitoring and emotional support.[19]

Parents are often surprised to hear that their influence can have so much impact. We hope that learning that you can play a major role in your child's choices is reassuring and inspiring, rather than a reason for guilt and self-blame. It is never too late to admit mistakes to children and model something different from what they have seen from you before.

Biological and Psychological Factors

Environment is never the whole story. Biology is also a factor. In early childhood, our brain's reward system matures, but the prefrontal cortex—the part of the brain that assesses situations more coolly and controls impulses and emotions—does not fully develop until we reach our midtwenties. Mental health professionals often use this helpful analogy: imagine the reward system as the gas pedal of a car and the prefrontal cortex as the brakes, except that in a teenager, the brakes are weak.[20] Drugs may do irreversible damage to the brain's ability to develop a good set of brakes. For example, cocaine can alter one's brain in such a way that encourages drug-seeking behavior.

There are also psychological factors to consider. Children who are highly impulsive and social, have previously exhibited risk-taking behaviors, and/or have been diagnosed with a psychiatric condition such as attention deficit/hyperactivity disorder (ADHD), oppositional defiant disorder (ODD), or conduct disorder are more susceptible.[21] These children often have something we call emotional dysregulation, which means their emotions mimic a roller coaster, with swift and extreme ups and downs. For these children, applying those "brakes" is much more difficult.

Conversely, children with anxiety and depression are more likely to turn to substances in an effort to manage their distress. Unfortunately, substance use is known to worsen both mood swings and anxiety, which in turn elevates the child's risk of a more severe and prolonged disorder.[22]

Many of these children also suffer from low self-esteem and social isolation, creating a domino effect of vulnerabilities.

What can parents do to prevent substance use disorders?

The key to prevention is to balance parental warmth and positive communication with parental monitoring. And the latter is exactly what it sounds like: knowing where your child is, what she is doing, who her friends are, and whether she is under the supervision of another responsible adult.[23] Here are a few other tips, most based on research, others on our clinical experience.[24, 25, 26, 27, 28, 29, 30, 31, 32]

- Don't normalize daily alcohol or cannabis use.
- Don't smoke cigarettes.
- Don't send mixed messages about substance use. For example, don't warn your children about the dangers of alcohol while simultaneously telling stories that portray excessive drinking as funny or inevitable. In our experience, these narratives are often gendered, with boys hearing more than girls that drinking to excess is an expected rite of passage.
- Try to make sure that your child is supervised after school and/or engaged in a sport or physical activity. For highly sociable children with a penchant for risk taking, enrolling them in an activity that gratifies both traits can be immensely helpful. Conversely, a child with social anxiety will learn strategies to manage his stress from activities such as debating or improv comedy.
- If it is part of your culture to have small amounts of alcohol at festive meals and you allow your child to participate, ensure that the amounts are minimal. Talk with your child about how moderation is expected.

- Know who your child's friends are. Be that annoying parent who confirms—by talking to other mothers and fathers—that parents are actually supervising during that sleepover or party.

- Don't buy your children alcohol or cannabis or offer them in your home before they and their friends are of legal age. Many parents think that it is safer for their children to drink and smoke at home than in public, but the older a child is before he starts to drink or use drugs, the less likely he is to develop a problem.

- Most important, make it clear to your child that she can always call you for help without fear of recrimination or anger. If she has drunk so much she is unwell or doesn't know where she is, make sure she knows to call you and that you will be there for her. She will have to explain her actions later, but in the moment, your priority will be to help her.

All of these recommendations support one of the central themes of this book: while not all mental illness is preventable, when possible, prevention is the most important thing you can do to help your kids decrease their risk of developing a serious mental health issue. Now let's return to Hussain, Saul, and Marcel, and see how they're faring.

Reaching a Diagnosis

It has been six long days since Saul and Hussain received that frightening Friday-night call. Forty-eight hours after Marcel's admission to the hospital, his liver enzymes had shot up, and he was showing signs of dangerously high levels of muscle breakdown. The doctors feared that his kidneys might fail, and he might require dialysis. His heart rate jumped erratically, and the hospital staff wondered if Marcel had taken "designer drugs" that their toxicology screen wouldn't necessarily have picked up. On the third day, Marcel finally woke up. Hussain didn't ask him about what happened, just hugged him and told him he loved him. Saul said very little.

Eventually Marcel confessed to the medical team that he thought he was taking Ecstasy the night of the party, but the doctors told Hussain and Saul that they suspect that it was cut with other drugs, perhaps phencyclidine (PCP, or angel dust). In short, Marcel is lucky to be alive, let alone medically stable. He has already discussed his substance use with Dr. Maria Ferroni, a pediatrician specializing in adolescent medicine, and has agreed to attend a substance use day program. Hussain and Saul are meeting with a social worker today in anticipation of Marcel's discharge later this afternoon.

Hussain is relieved about this appointment. He has been worrying about how they will keep Marcel safe at home after he leaves the hospital, and has lots of questions.

Tina Garcia, the social worker, offers Hussain and Saul a welcoming smile. "I have Dr. Ferroni's notes from her meetings with Marcel," she says. "Marcel is aware that I will be sharing some but not all of that discussion with you."

"We understand," Saul says.

Tina looks up from her notes. "As part of her assessment, Dr. Ferroni conducted something we call CRAFFT, which is a screening tool for substance use disorders in youth ages twelve to eighteen. Marcel and Dr. Ferroni agreed that I could share with you that Marcel scored very highly on the CRAFFT, which means he has a mixed substance use disorder and is in the most at-risk range."

She goes on to describe the screening test in more detail. CRAFFT is a mnemonic, and young patients are asked questions that reflect each letter:[33,34]

1. Have you ever driven in a **CAR** where the driver (possibly yourself) was drunk or high?

2. Do you ever use alcohol or drugs to **RELAX** or to feel better and to fit in?

3. Do you ever use alcohol or drugs when you are **ALONE**?

4. Do you ever **FORGET** things you did when you were using drugs or alcohol?

5. Do your **FAMILY** or **FRIENDS** ever tell you that you should cut down on your alcohol or drug use?

6. Have you ever gotten into **TROUBLE** when using alcohol or drugs?

As her words sink in, any hope Hussain had that Marcel's overdose was some sort of terrible one-off accident fades.

"I'd like to ask you some questions about Marcel's childhood and school life," Tina says.

As they answer the social worker's questions, Hussain realizes how busy he and Saul have been with their careers and the "business" of family life. They haven't taken much time to step back to think about Marcel's mental health. Has their busyness been an excuse? A way to avoid issues that have been increasingly uncomfortable in their own marriage, including disagreements about child rearing and their own coping styles?

"Marcel says most of his friends at school are heavy drug users. You may want to think about looking at somewhere else for him to go for the rest of the year. It will be hard for him to stay away from drugs in that peer group." Tina continues, "But just as important, Dr. Ferroni has suggested that we also talk about your own patterns with alcohol, given some comments that Marcel made to her about that."

Hussain feels Saul bristle beside him.

"I would like to make sure that Marcel is the focus here, not us," Saul says. "Isn't it more important for him to take responsibility for his own actions?"

"Of course," Tina says. "And that's a long-term goal. Right now we have to look at what's affecting him day to day and address that. The more involved you are, the greater his chances of overcoming this."

"What do you suggest we do?" Hussain asks. "We'll do anything to help Marcel recover."

"For starters, let's discuss the need for you to monitor him more closely, particularly when it comes to his phone and computer use. Many parents in our program hold on to their children's phones temporarily so they get some space from their daily habits and friends."

"Done," Hussain says immediately. Saul remains quiet.

"The day program we're enrolling Marcel in is very family focused, and in addition to working with you to support Marcel's recovery, you'll be asked to attend a parent education and support group once a week, and we'll conduct a family meeting every two weeks."

Saul clears his throat. "My schedule at the hospital is quite hectic. I may not be able to attend all the meetings."

"We have many parents with similar challenges," Tina replies. "We can work around your schedule."

"What are your outcomes like in the program?" Saul asks, his tone challenging.

"That's a great question." Tina looks thoughtful. "To be honest, our statistics are a bit spotty because we rely on the youth to respond to surveys that measure program outcomes, and the further out they are from discharge, the less likely they are to get back to us. But having said that, we know that many of them return to high school and graduate. They manage to use the skills they learn in the program to get to a level of functioning that is much better than when they joined us. Day programs may have an advantage over residential programs for youth with moderate substance use disorders because they force patients to deal with some of the real-life stressors that led to their drug use. We tend to reserve residential treatment for teens who can't get out from under their peer group and need some space to recover."

She pauses for a moment before looking Saul squarely in the face.

"We have an important window here. Marcel has agreed to attend the day program. Not all teens do. He'll need our team, you, friends, and family to support him so that he moves himself out of danger."

Later, in the car on the way home, as Saul drives, Hussain studies Marcel in the backseat. He looks younger and more rested than he has for months. He's gazing out the window rather than staring at his phone, which Hussain has in his pocket. Marcel had joined their meeting with Tina and agreed to discuss giving his parents access to his social media accounts before they return his phone to him. Instead of cutting off Marcel's relationships with his friends, they've agreed that, for now, his contact with them needs to be monitored. Hussain knows they aren't totally out of the woods, and it may take a while for him to get Saul to acknowledge their part in this—especially how they drink at home and why—but one thing at a time. Hussain feels confident that together, and with a bit of time, they can turn over a new leaf.

What are the treatments for substance use disorders?

Assessment: Medical, Psychological, and Family

The first step in a treatment plan is a thorough medical and psychological assessment. In most instances, a child's physician will check to see if there are any medical issues stemming from alcohol and drug use, such as sexually transmitted and/or blood-borne infections, and drug withdrawal.

The next steps are a psychological assessment with the adolescent, and then a family assessment to identify whether a youth is at risk of suicide and other psychiatric disorders apart from substance use. Many substance use treatment programs now include several types of health care professionals, so if your child also suffers from a mental illness, he will have an entire support team to help him address all his needs. Unlike Marcel, many adolescents don't acknowledge the extent of their problem right away, so obtaining a full history from family members in a second meeting can complete the picture.

At every stage of assessment, our goal is to gain the child's trust and to assess her interest in treatment. When we look at a teenager's level of openness to changing her behaviors, we rely on the following spectrum of readiness as we tailor treatment planning:[35]

- *precontemplation:* the person does not view himself as having a problem and therefore does not see a need for change;
- *contemplation:* the person acknowledges he has problems and considers the possibility of change;
- *determination:* the person makes the decision to pursue change and identifies and collects the resources he will need, for example, a smoker gets a nicotine patch from his nurse practitioner and signs up for a smoking cessation group that starts the following week;
- *action:* the person makes the desired changes;
- *maintenance:* the person incorporates the changes into his life for the foreseeable future; and
- *potential for relapse:* the person is unsuccessful, and the cycle begins again.

While it is helpful when a teen is motivated to pursue treatment, it is not required for treatment to be effective, contrary to what many parents believe. Family-based treatment for adolescents with substance use disorders has been demonstrated to be more effective than other types of treatment.[36] There is no evidence that any specific type of family work is best. It's simply familial support and engagement in the treatment process that is the effective ingredient.

When a child's life is at risk or the child has been found incapable of consenting to treatment, the law in most countries allows doctors and parents to intervene against his or her wishes. Because substance use disorders are usually only immediately life threatening during periods of acute intoxication, it can be difficult for parents to seek involuntary treatment outside these episodes, apart from some states and provinces that have additional laws that allow parents to intervene even if their child is out of immediate danger. That said, even where there are no such laws, we know from experience that parents have considerable power to persuade and influence, often more than they realize. Given the potentially irrevocable effects that heavy drug use has on an adolescent's brain—structural and functional brain changes that may contribute to increased impulsivity and reward-driven behaviors[37]—it's important that parents do everything in their power to get their children the help they need as early on in their disorder as possible.

Now we are going to turn to specific aspects of treatments—psychotherapies, harm reduction, and medication—so you can see what options are available to you and your child. We are strong proponents of the "wraparound" approach, which encourages parents to work with children and their care team to help adolescents reengage with the developmental tasks that have fallen by the wayside because of their substance use disorders. This includes building safe and healthy social and sexual relationships with peers, pursuing academic or vocational goals, engaging in healthy recreational activities, and reconnecting with family. These tasks require teens to manage interpersonal communication; develop good work habits; learn to tolerate frustration and boredom;

solve problems; and negotiate healthy boundaries with others. Helping adolescents acquire and practice these skills is a key aspect of treatment.[38]

As we alluded to in the social worker's discussion with Hussain and Saul, treatment can take place in a variety of settings. These include acute medical treatment for overdoses and withdrawal in hospital; outpatient treatment in either hospital or community clinics; day treatment programs; and residential programs, where the adolescent stays for several weeks or months in the facility, seeing her family during scheduled visits and therapy sessions. There isn't a great deal of specific research to help parents determine which treatment setting will be most beneficial to their child. Generally, health care professionals work with families to figure out which features of the child's disorder and which family factors are relevant. For example, an adolescent who has experienced many relapses during outpatient treatment because of ongoing proximity and contact with substance-using peers may find residential treatment more effective. Another teen who has had a relatively short-lived disorder and has strong family connections may benefit from those close ties and will do better with an outpatient or day treatment model. The adolescent's preference should also be taken into account, when safe to do so. Whatever the treatment model, rebuilding and maintaining family bonds is essential, given the importance of family connectedness as a positive prognostic factor in a child's recovery.

Psychotherapies

Cognitive behavior therapy (CBT) and motivational enhancement therapy (MET) are both used frequently as part of a wraparound approach.[39] The principles of CBT in treating substance use disorders are similar to those described in the previous chapter, with adaptations that focus on how the adolescent's thoughts and feelings shape his or her behavior with drugs.

MET is a nonconfrontational, collaborative approach that focuses on listening to the young person, asking clarifying questions, and building on the teen's aspirations to set treatment goals. MET complements theories of readiness to change, working to move children along the spectrum to action. In other words, MET is a way of engaging individuals with treatment rather than being a treatment on its own.[40]

Once you have established that the therapist is appropriately trained and accredited by their respective professional body (e.g., social work, psychology, psychotherapy, occupational therapy, nursing, medical psychotherapy, psychiatry) and confirmed with the health care professional who referred your child for therapy that the therapist has the relevant expertise, the personal qualities of the therapist are arguably as important as the type of therapy in determining whether your child will benefit from the therapy. A good therapist—one who is warm, genuine, and empathic, but also motivates and challenges your child—goes a long way. Start your search by asking your child's doctor for suggestions and referrals, as well as their school. Or visit your provincial or state professional associations for social work and psychology. Increasingly, there are regional websites and case navigation services (either online or by phone) that can direct parents to local and appropriate therapy and other mental health services. Sometimes your own employee assistance program may be able to refer you. We encourage you to find a therapist who engages with your child, but it may take time and perseverance to find the right fit. Tell your child at the outset that it may take meeting more than one therapist to find the right match.

Harm Reduction

If a child is willing to abstain from using substances, that is obviously a desirable goal to support, but if he refuses to stop, then we explore harm-reduction treatment approaches. In harm reduction, the goal becomes

the avoidance of harm from substance use, or use in moderation. Harm reduction may include abstinence from one or more substances but does not require it, and research has shown that not only can harm reduction reduce risk, but also it can build important treatment alliances that may prove lifesaving.[41, 42] Harm reduction may involve parents educating their child about the safety risks of her substance use (for example, driving after using cannabis) and agreeing on the consequences if their child doesn't adhere to their expectations for safe use, e.g., removing car privileges and/or reporting to her doctor if she does drive while high.

Medications

Young people with long-standing alcohol dependence may be offered benzodiazepines to manage withdrawal symptoms on an outpatient basis if a responsible adult is available to supervise them closely. If not, hospitalization would be considered carefully.[43] If a teen has a history of seizures, either during a previous withdrawal or from another medical cause, medically supervised management of withdrawal is recommended. The medications naltrexone (Revia, Vivitrol), acamprosate (Campral), and disulfiram (Antabuse) all have Health Canada approval and are effective in helping both to reduce alcohol use and to prevent relapse for adults with alcohol dependence,[44] and may be considered for children with moderate to severe versions of the same diagnosis under close medical supervision. None of these medications have Health Canada or FDA approval for their use in adolescents. However, alcohol dependence is a rare diagnosis for teenagers under the age of sixteen and remains relatively rare for teenagers in the sixteen-to-eighteen age group.

Adolescents who are opioid dependent may be offered buprenorphine (Subutex), a partial opioid agonist, for both detoxification and long-term stabilization, again with careful adult supervision and close monitoring by expert health care professionals. Methadone is a medication used as part of a treatment plan to treat opioid addiction that is itself an opioid. But it's used because it is longer acting than the short-acting and more addictive opioids such as heroin or oxycodone and therefore prevents withdrawal symptoms and reduces drug cravings, diminishing the negative effects of opioid misuse and allowing people who are addicted to opioids to rebuild their lives. Methadone is generally only used for maintenance treatment if buprenorphine and therapy have been unsuccessful.

Teenagers with substance use disorders are more likely than their healthy peers to smoke cigarettes, a dependence that comes with additional and severe health risks.[45] They should be offered nicotine replacement medications (available as skin patches, lozenges, gum, inhalers, and sprays) by their primary care physician to support them through withdrawal. For adolescents who have used these without success, physicians may consider either bupropion (Zyban, Wellbutrin) or varenicline (Chantix), two prescription medications that reduce nicotine cravings.[46] Both can have significant side effects, including new-onset suicidal ideation, so a discussion of potential benefits and risks with an informed health care professional is important.

Parents sometimes ask us about medical cannabinoids, strains of cannabis that contain little or none of the psychoactive component that produces the "high" associated with recreational use: tetrahydrocannabinol, or THC for short. Instead, they have more of a component called cannabidiol (CBD), which has little or no effect on a smoker's mental state. Given this, and the fact that medical cannabinoids are currently being explored in adults as a treatment for various psychiatric disorders, concerned mothers and fathers want to know whether substituting these for other forms of cannabis or other substances may help to moderate the potential harm. While there is some evidence suggesting a benefit from medical cannabinoids in certain medical disorders—such as chemotherapy-induced nausea in children undergoing treatment for cancer, and perhaps in the treatment of epilepsy—there is currently no robust evidence to suggest a benefit for any type of child and adolescent psychiatric disorder. In view of the known negative effects of recreational cannabis on developing brains, and the current lack of studies into the safety or effectiveness of medical cannabinoids for use in children and adolescents with psychiatric disorders, at this time we don't recommend medical cannabinoids for treatment of a substance use disorder or any other type of pediatric psychiatric disorder.

Navigating Setbacks

Three weeks after their initial consultation, Hussain and Saul are back in Tina's office for an emergency meeting after staff at the day program found a joint in Marcel's bag.

"I don't know why it was there," Marcel says. "I wasn't going to smoke it during program."

Tina sits back in her chair. "I'm happy to hear that, Marcel, given the negative impact that would have on not just your recovery but on the other kids in the program. But smoking outside the program also has an impact, and we need to talk about that."

Marcel straightens in his seat, an angry look on his face. "Everyone here keeps saying we're a community and our behavior impacts everyone else. But my dads don't believe that. Each individual is responsible for their own choices."

Hussain interjects, "Marcel, that's not true. We've told you many times that we're here to support you."

"Then why is Pa still drinking every night? I'm not an idiot. I smell it on him. I see when he's tuned out." Marcel's voice rises. "What do you think that's like for me?"

Saul, who indeed has seemed tuned out for most of the meeting, raises his own voice in response. "We're here to talk about you! I'm an adult, and I can manage my own behavior. You're a kid who's messed up, which is why we are here."

Marcel gets up and leaves, slamming the door behind him.

Tina picks up her phone and murmurs something into it before she turns back to Hussain and Saul. "Our child and youth counsellor is going to make sure Marcel's okay."

Hussain looks over at Saul. "I would say the ball's in your court."

Saul addresses Tina. "Hussain has asked me a number of times to cut down on my drinking and to stop drinking entirely during the week, but I see it as pandering to Marcel. Hussain says I'm rationalizing, but I don't agree."

"Saul, your substance use has been a recurring theme in Marcel's treatment, but it seems we may have hit a wall," Tina says. "I'm going to ask you and Hussain to talk on your own and think about how we can move forward."

Hussain leans over and takes his husband's hand. "We need to do absolutely everything to help him, Saul. Absolutely everything. He's telling us what he needs. We can do this—together."

What happens when a child relapses?

Marcel's relapse is not uncommon, and because of that, we caution parents that more than one period of treatment may be needed. We typically begin with the adolescent's preference and the least disruptive and restrictive option—usually outpatient, with appointments once or twice a week, or day treatment—and move to more intensive residential models if initial treatments are not successful. We never change treatments lightly and make sure that any decision is based on the underlying reasons for the child's setback.

Parents often ask us about "tough love" approaches in which a child is barred from the home if he or she uses drugs. The fact is that homeless children living on the street are at a higher risk of more severe substance use disorders, as well as overdosing, being assaulted, attempting suicide—and dying—so, needless to say, this should be avoided at all costs.[47, 48] First, we recommend that parents discuss clear expectations for treatment and behavior with their child and then, together, agree on a timeline and consequences if he or she fails to meet those expectations. Sometimes, though, the child's presence jeopardizes the well-being and safety of other family members. Under such circumstances, having him leave the home temporarily is a reasonable course of action. However, trying to provide a realistic treatment option or assisting with other relatively safe housing options—such as living with a relative—is generally preferable to expelling a child from the home, particularly in anger. We encourage parents to tell their child that he will always be welcome back if he can guarantee safety for others and is willing to engage in treatment.

We advocate for parents' taking the long view and not seeing today's failure as evidence that all is hopeless. Time and love, even at a partial distance, can be very powerful contributors to recovery.

After Treatment

Marcel did not complete day treatment and suffered another serious overdose. But after that, he agreed to an eight-month stay in residential treatment. Since leaving the facility, he has remained involved in individual and group therapy and has now been drug free for a full year. He is back in a new alternative school, where the teachers know his history and have been supportive.

In addition to attending a parent group once a month, Hussain and Saul have made a point of joining their son in activities he loves. Saul and Marcel now have a weekly basketball date, and Hussain and Marcel are taking Spanish together. They've also made an effort to get to know Marcel's friends and their parents, and they are scrupulous about keeping track of where Marcel is at all times.

Saul, meanwhile, enrolled in a harm reduction program for his alcohol use, during which he identified what he saw as risks of his current drinking patterns—most importantly, their impact on Marcel. He also reviewed medically established healthy drinking guidelines and set goals for himself to reduce his weekly intake. His work in the program led to a referral for therapy, which he pursued reluctantly with Hussain's encouragement. He now admits that both experiences opened his eyes to how his own father's drinking and beliefs about manliness and alcohol intake impacted his habits. He has found healthier coping strategies for the stress he feels from work. Saul and Hussain restrict their drinking to weekends and have imposed strict limits on quantity.

At their check-in with Tina, she says, "You three impress me."

"Why?" Marcel asks.

She flashes them her characteristic warm smile. "When you first came to me, you weren't functioning as a family support team, and you weren't honest with yourselves or with one another. Now you are. It's not that all the challenges are behind you, but you're working together, and you admit when there are setbacks."

Marcel is seated between his fathers. When they join hands, he adds his own on top.

"We're a family," Marcel says. "Isn't that what we're supposed to do?"

Eating Disorders

A Child in Distress

Anita and Sanjay and their son Ravi sit in the waiting room of their local hospital's psychiatry urgent care clinic. Ravi, who is fourteen, is huddled in a large hoodie on a vinyl-covered bench across from his parents, his body folded over his phone. He is holding a half-eaten apple, the remains of the meager breakfast that Anita cajoled him into having.

Until recently, the Mehtas' middle son had been an avid eater with a solid, muscular build. He was a gregarious, happy, hardworking boy whom teachers described as a pleasure to have in their class. Anita and Sanjay often privately referred to Ravi as their "easy" child.

Then, during a routine checkup last spring, Ravi's pediatrician told them that their son was getting into the higher range of body mass index (BMI) percentiles for his age. She explained that BMI is calculated using a child's height and weight, but unlike in adults, an absolute BMI number in children is less relevant than how the child's BMI compares with other children of the same age. Ravi's BMI-for-age was 75, meaning that his weight was greater than 75 percent of other children's of the same age and sex. The pediatrician reminded them that BMIs don't take into account different builds and degrees of muscularity, but she still cautioned them to be careful with Ravi's diet.

"This is nonsense," Sanjay said to Anita after the appointment.

She wasn't so sure. "Maybe the doctor has a point. It wouldn't hurt for our whole family to cut down on pop and sweet desserts, and to eat better in general."

Unlike his older sister, Najma, and his younger brother, Gaurev, who both loudly scorned this plan, Ravi endorsed it enthusiastically, cutting out fatty foods and carbohydrates, and turning to protein shakes, tofu, fruit, and vegetables. He started running every morning and going to the gym at his school several times a week, in addition to his hockey and baseball teams' practices and games. At first, Anita and Sanjay congratulated Ravi on his drive, but then they began to notice a drastic change in their son's weight and attitude. Since that checkup ten months ago, Ravi has lost 35 pounds, dropping from 170 to 135, or approximately 20 percent of his body weight, and he has become withdrawn, irritable, and glum.

Anita and Sanjay talked to him about easing up on his diet and exercise but did not consider his behavior to be a serious problem. After all, their other two children have eating issues: Gaurev is a picky eater, and Najma cycles through various popular diets, breaking them within a few days, complaining that she is starving. Both children weather these issues unscathed. Anita and Sanjay had been sure Ravi would, too, until a week ago when, during his hockey game, Ravi left the ice, telling his coach he felt dizzy and light-headed. The coach advised them to bring him to the hospital's emergency department straightaway.

On the car ride to the hospital, Sanjay tried to comfort Anita. "You know how careful the coaches and trainers are these days. They're all worried about liability."

But they did not get the reassurance they were hoping for from the emergency room doctor. After examining Ravi and ordering some blood tests, she said, "Ravi can go home, but I'm worried about his weight loss. I want to refer him to the hospital's psychiatry urgent care clinic to rule out an eating disorder."

Sanjay and Anita were shocked. An eating disorder? How could this be? Ravi had simply succeeded at what everyone tries to do: eat more healthily and lose some weight. Yes, he had taken it a bit too far, but surely he didn't have an eating disorder. Wasn't that a diagnosis for dangerously skinny young girls who wanted to look like fashion models? The Mehtas said nothing to each other as they drove Ravi home and then gave him a light supper and fluids, as instructed by the doctor. For the first time in months, Ravi ate their choice of food without protest and answered their inquiries with one-word replies.

Later, in bed that night, Anita sobbed in Sanjay's arms. "Do you think our son really has an eating disorder? I feel so stupid, like such a bad mother."

"You are a great mother," Sanjay said soothingly. "I'm the one who told him how proud I was that he was taking charge of his fitness. I kept complimenting him every time he ordered a salad instead of a burger and fries. I never expected something like this from Ravi." He took Anita's hand. "Let's try to stay calm. We don't know what the issue is yet."

But Anita shook her head. "Remember when Najma and I used to tease him for having a round tummy? Maybe he didn't realize it was just fun, just silliness. Maybe I caused this?"

What is an eating disorder?

Anita and Sanjay are correct in recognizing that not every child who changes his eating patterns has an eating disorder. It is not unusual for some children transitioning from half days of kindergarten to full days of school to eat little or nothing at lunch because they are too distracted by their friends and the need to get out to the playground. Similarly, students transitioning to high school in a location where they need to travel farther in the mornings may stop eating breakfast at home in order to stay in bed until the last possible moment, barely eat lunch, and then "graze," eating snacks from the time they get home until they go to bed. As children grow up, their relationship with food and their bodies may change in ways that are not necessarily cause for concern. However, if their eating behavior and weight changes drastically, these are warning signs that any prior fussiness about food or sporadic dissatisfaction with their bodies has moved into the realm of a serious eating disorder.

An eating disorder is a potentially life-threatening illness that causes significant disruption in eating and related thoughts and emotions, resulting in serious negative medical and psychological impacts, including destructive thoughts and feelings about body image and/or food, such as feeling exceptionally unattractive and overweight despite being at or below a healthy weight.[1]

Dieting is one of the most common gateways to an eating disorder. Health care professionals increasingly discourage dieting, as the evidence of its harms for adults, and especially for children and adolescents, becomes clearer. Dieting can negatively affect academic performance, self-esteem, energy, sleep, bone density, and, ironically, can lead to weight gain over time. We know that 50 percent of teenage girls and 25 percent of teenage boys will try to lose weight intentionally.[2] Fortunately, only a small minority of these children will go on to have an eating disorder, but parents should be vigilant if confronted with a dieting child.

How common are eating disorders? US statistics put an adolescent's risk of developing an eating disorder at 2.7 percent, with eating disorders twice as prevalent in females than in males, and their overall prevalence increasing slightly with age.[3] Although we don't have current robust child statistics in Canada, an older study estimated that 1.5 percent of Canadian women had an eating disorder at any given time, but this number—which may be higher by now—doesn't include individuals with disordered eating who don't fit neatly into a diagnostic category: for example, someone who yo-yo diets, feels terrible about her weight despite being healthy, and sometimes overeats and vomits after eating but not on a regular basis.[4] What these numbers don't convey is the potential lethality of eating disorders, which have the highest mortality rate of all mental illnesses, with deaths resulting from both medical complications and high suicide rates.[5]

We emphasize these tragic facts to counter the widely held but dangerously inaccurate misperception that eating disorders are strictly a teenage girl phenomenon; "a phase" that young people will outgrow on their own. In recent years, the demographics of who develops an eating disorder have changed: all types of eating disorders have been increasingly identified in younger children, in boys, and in children from minority groups.[6]

What are the different types of eating disorders and their warning signs?

We know that it can be challenging for parents to identify whether a child's eating behavior has crossed the line into danger. Given that, we've outlined the four most common eating disorders and their specific warning signs below, so that if your child exhibits any of these behaviors, you will know to intervene early.

Anorexia Nervosa

You've likely heard of this disease, as it is the most well-known eating disorder. Anorexia nervosa is a psychiatric disorder that causes the sufferer to eat less and less food because of an intense fear of gaining weight or becoming fat. What you may not know is that there are two types of anorexia nervosa: restricting and binge-eating/purging. The primary symptom of the restricting type is eating minimally and exercising excessively. By contrast, a person suffering from the binge-eating/purging type alternates between eating almost nothing and consuming extremely large amounts of food, which she then attempts to purge through vomiting or taking laxatives or other medicines. Both forms are linked to significant weight loss, which leads to an unhealthily low body weight.

Anita and Sanjay noticed several months ago that Ravi was cutting his food into smaller and smaller pieces. What's more, he would move it around on his plate or hide it under his napkin, avoid foods he once loved, and become angry when questioned about his food choices. These are all early warning signs that something is wrong. So is Ravi's rigid exercise regimen. The hours he spends on physical activity every day make it hard for him to see his friends, to have downtime, and to get to bed at a decent hour. Like Ravi, children in the beginning stages of this illness often describe an experience of increased focus, energy, and euphoria. However, as their bodies become increasingly malnourished, their energy drops, their memory and concentration worsen, and their grades start to fall. Emotionally, they become withdrawn, moody, preoccupied, and anxious, but the physical toll is even more severe: heart rate and bowels slow down, blood pressure and body temperature drop, girls stop menstruating, and scalp hair falls out, while fine, downy hair called lanugo begins to cover the body.

As parents, one of the most difficult and mysterious aspects of anorexia nervosa is how distorted a child's perception of her body becomes and how dissatisfied she is with her body. Even if the disease has progressed so far that the child is emaciated, the image she sees reflected in a mirror shows body parts that are unacceptably large or fat, with only rare glimpses of her body's gaunt reality.

If the disease is left untreated, sufferers become at serious risk of drug and alcohol abuse, suicide attempts, and multi-organ failure. That is why it is so important that parents are aware of early warning signs. Getting help early on improves recovery significantly and lessens the chance of the disease progressing to these more advanced, dangerous stages.[7]

Bulimia Nervosa

The second most widely known eating disorder is bulimia nervosa. Those who suffer from it regularly eat large amounts of food very quickly and then desperately try to get rid of calories by vomiting, misusing medicines, exercising excessively, or fasting. However, unlike the binge/purge version of anorexia nervosa, bulimia is not associated with significant weight loss. It can be more difficult to detect if a child is struggling when he or she is at an average or above-average weight and doesn't look visibly unwell in the early stages of the illness.

There *are* some telltale signs parents can watch for, though, such as bathroom visits during or immediately after meals, sores on their children's knuckles (from inserting them down their throat to cause vomiting), and, over time, swelling around the jawline caused by inflamed salivary glands, and tooth decay from the acid in vomit that erodes tooth enamel. In fact, dentists are sometimes the first health care professionals to diagnose purging behaviors.

As with anorexia, bulimic children generally see themselves as larger than they are and worry excessively that they are fat.[8] They frequently hide their bodies in baggy clothing, avoid wearing swimsuits, or spend a significant amount of time getting ready or changing their clothes. Other warning signs include food missing from the kitchen and sometimes missing money that the child has taken surreptitiously to buy food.

Avoidant/Restrictive Food Intake Disorder (ARFID)

This eating disorder is not as well known as others, partially because of its cumbersome label, and partially because it is often confused with picky eating, but 5 percent to 20 percent of children we see for intensive eating disorder treatment suffer from ARFID. It's a serious illness in which the child doesn't eat enough to meet his nutritional and/or energy needs, and the subsequent malnutrition can cause unhealthy weight loss or growth delays.

Children with ARFID are often disinterested in food, need reminders to eat, and complain about not liking the textures, look, smell, and taste of food. This kind of fussiness can be normal for some young kids, and most grow out of it, but some don't. It is the latter group of children who are at risk of developing ARFID. We don't yet know why some boys and girls with fussy eating habits develop ARFID and others do not, but research suggests that children with anxiety, autism spectrum disorder, and learning disorders are more susceptible.

If you are the parent of a fussy eater and aren't sure if the problem is more serious, ask your child's doctor about whether he is staying on his growth curve. (These are the charts of your child's height and weight that his health care provider checks regularly.) Healthy children tend to stick pretty closely to their growth curves, so if your child has always been in the 25th percentile for height and the 50th percentile for weight, you should expect him to stay there. And it's a good sign if his blood tests show that he is meeting his nutritional needs (iron, calcium, vitamin B_{12}). You should worry only if his eating patterns are inhibiting normal physical growth and development or the important development tasks of childhood, such as socializing with other children or eating outside the home.

Binge-Eating Disorder

Anorexia, bulimia, and binge-eating disorder all share similar risk factors: family history, a personal history of dieting, prior trauma, experiences of food insecurity or of food being overused as a reward or soother. However, binge-eating disorder manifests a little differently from the other two. A child suffering from binge-eating disorder will frequently overeat, usually when she's alone, because of feelings of self-disgust, guilt, and embarrassment. Unlike a child with anorexia nervosa or bulimia, she doesn't try to get rid of food or calories. As a result, she is often, but not always, above her naturally expected weight. These children usually perceive their body size accurately.

As parents, we know that it can be challenging to discern if your child is binging or eating erratically because she needs the nutrition as she hasn't eaten enough earlier in the day or if there is something more serious going on. This is particularly true during your child's adolescent growth spurts. If you are concerned, ask yourself if your child frequently eats alone and, despite denying unusual eating patterns, is increasingly gaining weight. Consider if there are other emotional or psychological factors that may contribute to compulsive overeating. It can be difficult for children and adolescents struggling with binge-eating to acknowledge their symptoms, given their shame and guilt, which can leave parents and clinicians trying to analyze the discrepancy between what they say and what they do.

Despite the variation between different types of eating disorders, there are some key overlapping warning signs that parents can look for: namely, sustained changes in eating patterns, exercise, and weight. If your child exhibits these signs, it is important to seek treatment for them as soon as possible. As with anorexia nervosa, early intervention will significantly increase your child's chance of recovery.

If you are concerned, but there hasn't been a moment of crisis as in Ravi's story, the first step is to contact your family doctor and schedule a medical checkup for your child. Let the physician know ahead of time what has you worried and why. If your doctor confirms that there is a problem, he or she will likely refer your child to a health care professional with expertise in assessing and treating eating disorders, which is how Ravi and his parents got to the urgent care psychiatry clinic. After we review the risk factors that may increase your child's likelihood of developing an eating disorder, we will return to our story to see how Ravi's assessment goes.

What are the risk factors for developing an eating disorder?

Environmental Factors

When it comes to the environmental risk factors for developing an eating disorder, the most important thing to consider is which foods and body images our children learn are healthy, and that starts with us, their parents.

We all question what's best for our children, and with the rising rates of childhood obesity, we often ask ourselves what's too much food, what's not enough, and what's just right. First, we have to address our own relationships with food and weight, because our eating habits and attitudes set the stage for our children's. Growing up, many of us heard, "Finish what's on your plate." Or "Don't waste food. Think about all the children who are starving." Or we were asked, "Do you really need a second helping?" Perhaps you have even repeated a version of these statements to your own children. The problem with these kinds of comments is that they damage the natural relationship we have to our appetites. In other words, they stop us from listening to what our bodies are telling us they need and encourage us to either overeat or undereat.

To make matters worse for parents, we are often besieged by contradictory advice on how to feed our kids. Say no to sweets; say yes to sweets because depriving kids causes overeating. Don't worry about picky eating, they'll grow out of it; do worry about picky eating, as it leads to poor nutrition. Most of us struggle to find time to shop for and prepare nutritious meals so, out of guilt, we cut corners and give in to our children's demands to give them only foods they like. Teaching a child to enjoy food textures and flavors takes time, and since we are busier than ever before, it is easy to think that some food—even if we know it is not what we should be providing—is better than none.

And parents can control only so much of what their kids learn about healthy eating and physical activity. These days, children come home with questions and recommendations from their schools. While some of what is taught is valuable—such as the emphasis on the benefits of physical activity—some prevention programs have had the unanticipated and unwanted effect of providing vulnerable children with ideas about how to lose weight.[9] The truth is, unless a doctor says a child's weight is compromising his or her health, dieting and weight loss should not be recommended. If a doctor does recommend losing weight, any changes to your child's diet should be made under close medical supervision.

Exposing children to negative comments about above-average weights and shapes and focusing on restrictive diets can contribute to an unhealthy body image and disordered eating.[10, 11, 12] Things that parents say to—or in earshot of—children can lead them to think they should be dieting and losing weight. For example, the daughter who hears her mother bemoan a few pounds of weight gain after a holiday or the son who hears his father refer to a colleague as unhealthily fat may question how their own bodies fit with their parents' ideas of what is healthy and attractive.

The good news is that when parents become aware of the potential negative impact of their words, they can reverse course and teach themselves and their children that appropriate amounts of physical activity are the best way to maintain good health. Of course, some forms of exercise are better than others. Team sports are good experiences for most children because they combine fun, experiences of mastery and frustration, and lessons in the challenges and value of teamwork. The culture in some sports—such as dancing, gymnastics, figure skating, and competitive swimming[13]—has historically encouraged dieting and rewarded thinness, and has been linked to higher rates of eating disorders. If your child has a passion for one of these sports, don't necessarily discourage his or her participation but be vigilant about the approach his or her coaches and teammates take to eating and weight loss. Consider your child's temperament and body image and other risk factors before proceeding.

Sex and gender identity also play roles in determining a child's likelihood of developing an eating disorder. Girls are far more likely to develop problems with their eating, which is why Anita and Sanjay found it hard to believe that their son might have an eating disorder. That being said, the number of young boys diagnosed with eating disorders has increased significantly in the past two decades, reflecting a substantial societal change in how weight and appearance are valued for both sexes.[14] There is also evidence that children with sexual minority orientations (homosexual, bisexual, or pansexual), transgender and nonbinary identities (those who identify as neither male nor female), and particularly sex-assigned females at birth who identify as male are at increased risk of developing eating disorders.[15, 16]

We include these references to sex and gender as environmental factors, although there may be biological contributors at work here, as there is historical evidence that the differential exposure to the so-called thin ideal among women, in contrast to males, has a strong negative effect on women's body image and self-esteem, and is related to increased rates of anxious and depressive symptoms,[17] all risk factors for disordered eating. As the thin ideal has spread to non-Western parts of the world, so have rates of eating disorders in those countries.[18] Within the transgender community, research has demonstrated that many trans males and females similarly wish to achieve idealized body images for their identified gender.[19]

Biological and Psychological Factors

One of the most common questions parents ask us is why some children, even within the same family, are immune to the environmental influences we have just outlined, while others absorb and act upon negative messages around food and develop eating disorders. In most cases, it comes down to biology—a child's genetically determined cluster of characteristics—and personality traits that are partially determined by genetics.

When it comes to genetic vulnerability, we now know that eating disorders, particularly anorexia nervosa, run in families, with relatives of individuals with eating disorders seven to twelve times more likely to develop an eating disorder.[20] Cynthia Bulik, a well-known researcher in the field, said, "Genes load the gun, and the environment pulls the trigger."[21] In other words, if your family has a history of eating disorders, and your child is involved in an aesthetic sport such as gymnastics, she has an elevated risk of developing an eating disorder.

Medical illness is also a factor. For example, young women with diabetes have approximately twice the risk of developing eating disorders as girls of the same age without diabetes. This is likely because those with diabetes have an increased focus on food and are more likely to experience unwanted weight changes because of their treatment.

We know that certain personality traits may contribute to a child's vulnerability to an eating disorder. Children who are shy, inhibited, perfectionistic, and have a capacity for perseverance are more at risk of developing anorexia nervosa. So are those with social anxiety and obsessive-compulsive disorder. Children who are impulsive, undergo early puberty, have diagnoses of ADHD,[22, 23] and experience challenges managing their emotions are more prone to bulimia. These risk factors can cause children to develop dissatisfaction with their bodies and try to lose weight through disordered eating.

As parents ourselves, we understand that this information is daunting, but remember, not all children with some or any of these predisposing factors develop eating disorders. The takeaway here is that being aware of the risks—environmental, biological, and psychological—allows you to intervene early to help prevent your child from developing an eating disorder. We will talk more about the specific ways you can do so below.

What can parents do to prevent eating disorders?

Preventing eating disorders is always easier than treating them. While certain risk factors are out of our control, there are a few things we can do as parents to encourage healthy approaches to eating, exercise, and body image in our children. Here are some practical tips drawn from our clinical experience and the findings of researchers in the field:

- Offer younger children structured food choices that include a variety of foods from each food group, with different tastes, textures, and colors.[24] And when it comes to who is in charge of what, as one authority has put it, your job as parents is to decide which foods are offered, and when and where; it's up to your children to decide which food to eat and how much.[25]

- If your child is particularly picky, keep in mind that some children may need to try a new food ten or more times before they accept it, so don't give up. Give your child at least one food you know he likes, but offer the same food as the rest of the family and expect him to eat it.

- Encourage children to follow their appetite cues. Avoid distractions at the dinner table and don't push children to finish what is on their plates if they say they are full.
- Ensure that the majority of your family's diet is nutritional, unprocessed foods, but try not to ban foods that are relatively less nutritious. Instead, present them regularly in small amounts and when your children are not excessively hungry.
- Don't describe foods as good or bad. Use terms such as "growing food" and "fun food."[26]
- Avoid keeping sugary drinks at home for regular consumption.
- Make sure children get daily physical activity.
- Show children that exercise is fun and a good way to interact with other people by role modeling that behavior yourself.
- Avoid making pejorative comments regarding your own, your child's, or other people's weight and shape.
- Limit children's screen time and encourage adequate sleep.

If you recognize that your child's weight is naturally higher than that of other children his or her age, it's best to avoid any type of dietary restrictions. Instead, focus on regular physical activity, a positive body image that focuses on strength and health, and good nutrition. This approach will help your child avoid the yo-yo dieting and body shame that are counterproductive to achieving a healthy, stable weight and body image.

That isn't to say that some children won't require more help. Those who are morbidly obese, have medical issues, or eat in a self-destructive pattern stemming from emotional distress, boredom, or habit will likely require professional intervention. Even in these situations, however, experts agree that engaging your family to change environmental factors—such as physical activity, sleep, and food choices—will lead to greater success and have far fewer risks than restricting a child's food intake.

Remember, too, that you can do everything right as a parent, but given all the other relevant variables, your child may still develop an eating disorder. It happens. In those instances, the important thing is to recognize that your child is struggling and to get her the help she needs.

Reaching a Diagnosis

After the child psychiatrist, Dr. Andrea Monarch, and the nurse practitioner who works with her, Melanie Wang, introduce themselves to Anita, Sanjay, and Ravi, they all gather in Dr. Monarch's office. As Nurse Wang asks Ravi about his sports teams, school, and other interests, Sanjay notices his son's shoulders relax, which is when the nurse switches gears.

"Ravi, the emergency doctor asked us to help you and your parents figure out if you have an eating disorder, and to talk about what to do if that's the case. Does that fit with what you thought we would be discussing today?"

Sanjay takes Anita's hand without looking at her, not wanting to upset his own fragile equilibrium by seeing her expression. The silence feels endless until Ravi breaks it with a sound barely louder than a sigh.

"Yes."

"Good. I'll need to ask you about your eating, physical activity, and thoughts and feelings about your body. Would this next part be easier to talk about on your own?"

"Yes," Ravi says again.

"While we're at it, I'm going to check your weight, blood pressure, heart rate—all the things they did in the emergency department—just to see where we are at," Nurse Wang says kindly. "I'm also going to grab you a milk and a snack."

Although his son was given a choice about the context of the next part of the interview, Sanjay notes that the physical exam and snack are presented as inevitable. Given Ravi's reluctance to eat anything he is told to, he is curious how these two things will go. As he watches Ravi's thin frame moving out of the office, Sanjay fights an urge to leap up, grab his son, and take him home, as if they could go back to a time when Ravi was happy, before the words *eating disorder*.

Once Ravi and the nurse have left, Dr. Monarch turns to Sanjay and Anita. "Mr. and Ms. Mehta," she begins, "we are reasonably confident from reviewing the emergency department notes that Ravi is struggling with anorexia nervosa, restricting type, which means he's restricting his food intake and overexercising. There don't appear to be any purging behaviors, but these tend to be the symptoms patients hide, so today we'll try to confirm with a thorough physical exam and blood tests that Ravi's illness hasn't progressed that far."

Tears well up in Anita's eyes. "I'm feeling overwhelmed," she says. "I can't believe we allowed Ravi to get to a place where he is in physical danger. You must think we're terrible parents."

Dr. Monarch offers her a box of tissues. "Ms. Mehta, most parents feel the same way you do, but you can help your son much more than you think. After this morning, we'll have a much better sense of what's going on with Ravi and how open he is to treatment. Of course, if it's not medically safe to manage his condition outside the hospital, we'll bring him in, but even if we do, he'll be coming home to you as soon as possible for the rest of his treatment."

"I appreciate your confidence in us, Doctor," Sanjay says. "What we need, though, is a foolproof system to help our son."

Dr. Monarch smiles. "I'm afraid there's no such system, but what works is a collaborative effort. We'll work with you and teach you how to best help Ravi. Over the next while, you'll need to supervise all his meals;

choose what he eats instead of allowing him to pick; ensure he finishes what you give him; support him after meals, as he'll likely feel panicked and uncomfortable; and watch that he doesn't overexercise."

Sanjay turns to Anita. "I think we can do this. We've been trying to cajole Ravi, but it hasn't been working. We need to take charge and make sure he does what he needs to do to be healthy. Right, Doctor?"

"Right," Dr. Monarch agrees. "This can be a long road, and there may be more emergency department visits. That's just the nature of this illness and the recovery process. We understand that a seriously ill child is every parent's worst fear and the two of you are under huge stress, but you will also have a team here for you."

Anita rests a hand on Sanjay's forearm.

Dr. Monarch moves on. "Do either of you have a family history of eating disorders? Depression or anxiety? Alcoholism or drug abuse?"

Anita explains that her family are all in India, where mental illness isn't talked about much. She does remember her mother being highly anxious and having some very strange eating habits. Her sister, Nandiya, is a marathon runner and exceptionally thin, to the extent that she had difficulty becoming pregnant and her doctor told her she needed to gain weight. Sanjay adds that his father is a bit of a hypochondriac, one of his older brother drinks heavily, and his younger sister received treatment for postpartum depression.

"Has anyone in the family made a suicide attempt?"

The question hangs in the air for a moment before they shake their heads. Neither Sanjay nor Anita have said the word *suicide* out loud to one another, but Ravi's withdrawal has frightened them, and they've both wondered if he is at risk. It's a thought that neither of them can bear to contemplate for more than a second.

"Have you worried about Ravi hurting himself?"

Anita's tears well up again. "Yes, particularly when he stopped wanting to see his friends, sit with us after dinner, or watch hockey games with Sanjay and his brother on weekends, which used to be a big treat."

"But he's never said anything," Sanjay says. "Not outright."

Dr. Monarch proceeds to ask about Anita's pregnancies, Ravi's delivery, his early eating habits, developmental milestones, his transition to kindergarten and first grade, and how he related to other children and unfamiliar adults.

Sanjay and Anita tell her about Ravi's childhood habits—lining up his toys every night, making lists the night before of what he needed for school the next day, ensuring that his clothes matched—and his distress whenever he brought home a grade that was less than stellar.

"Any other ritualistic and repetitive behaviors?"

Sanjay and Anita recollect Ravi checking his ears multiple times a day at age five or so after seeing the animated film *Pinocchio*.

"Do you remember he wouldn't tell us what was wrong, until one night he broke down and burst into tears and said he was worried he was growing donkey ears?" Sanjay asks Anita, who nods.

"It doesn't sound like Ravi has obsessive-compulsive disorder, but he may have obsessive-compulsive traits and behaviors, which put him at risk for an eating disorder, because he always wants to do his best—in this case, with so-called healthy eating and exercise," Dr. Monarch explains. She adds that these traits are inherited and overlap in families. "In fact, many of us in medicine have these behaviors." She grins. "The attention to detail, rule following, conscientiousness, desire to do one's best—these aren't bad things. They just need to be managed."

Sanjay smiles back at the doctor. He sees something of himself in what she has just said.

Just then, Nurse Wang and Ravi reenter the room.

"I've repeated Ravi's vital signs," the nurse says. "They were consistent with what we saw in his emergency department visit, and he's had a bran muffin and a large milk. We had a chat about what Ravi will need to change at home for us to feel he can be safe as an outpatient for now, and he feels he can work with his parents to increase his food intake." She looks at Ravi encouragingly. "He knows it's going to be hard, but he wants to try if his parents agree."

Sanjay and Anita exchange a glance. Ravi hasn't eaten a muffin in months, complaining they contain too much fat, nor drunk any milk apart from small amounts of skim.

Dr. Monarch turns to Ravi. "The heart tracing we have for you and your blood work from your emergency department visit are okay, and the fact that your blood pressure and heart rate today are stable and you ate the snack we gave you are good signs."

Ravi seems relieved. "Does that mean I don't need to come into the hospital?"

"As long as your parents feel confident that you can make the changes you need to at home—with their support, of course—we don't think you need to come in. Nurse Wang and I are going to discuss your status with our eating disorders team and ask them to continue treating you as an outpatient. That means you'll be working with their team on your health and relationships to food and your body."

Neither Sanjay nor Anita knows if they will be able to change the patterns between them and Ravi that led them here, but the visit has offered them comfort, and they feel reassured knowing the hospital team will be there to support them if they run into more trouble.

Dr. Monarch explains to Ravi that she and the nurse practitioner can confirm based on his emergency department assessment and their interviews with him and his parents that he has anorexia nervosa. He doesn't respond, but both Sanjay and Anita notice that he doesn't seem surprised. Dr. Monarch reiterates what Nurse Wang has already told him: that to remain an outpatient, he will need to eat what his parents give him and to take a break from vigorous exercise. "Your body, particularly your heart, needs a rest. It will be difficult for you to believe that your parents are giving you the right amount of food because your eating disorder will try to persuade you that it's too much and that putting on weight isn't healthy for you, but you need to trust us more than the eating disorder."

Ravi nods. "It's weird. When I talked to Nurse Wang, it was like she knew what's been going on in my head. I have these thoughts, like, 'It's too much food,' and then, 'No, it's not, you need it.' Or 'Ravi, don't be such a wimp; you're supposed to run every day.' I feel so tired all the time. I just don't know what's been going on, so, like, what you're saying, it's . . . scary . . . but I feel kinda . . ."

"Kind of what?" Dr. Monarch asks.

"Well, like, I feel a bit more hopeful. Even though I know I'm not going to like it when my parents make me eat a whole lunch and stuff."

"You will need to eat more than you want to," Dr. Monarch acknowledges. "But we won't be pushing too hard at the beginning. It's better for your body to get used to a healthy amount of food again gradually. It will get easier with time."

Ravi looks both dubious and hopeful. Anita puts her arm around him, and he doesn't shrug it off.

Dr. Monarch and Nurse Wang wrap up, providing Anita and Sanjay with written instructions for next steps and letting them know they will be hearing from the eating disorders clinic within the next two weeks. They both shake each family member's hand and usher them out of the room.

What are the treatments for eating disorders?

As we saw in the above vignette, Ravi's health care providers diagnosed him with anorexia nervosa, but first, they confirmed he was medically stable and performed a thorough medical assessment to rule out other possible causes for his changes in eating and weight, such as celiac disease (an abnormal immune response in the gut to foods containing gluten), inflammatory bowel disease (chronic inflammation of the gastrointestinal tract leading to damage), or lactose intolerance (an enzyme deficiency that prevents breakdown of lactose in cow's milk products, causing gastrointestinal discomfort and symptoms). This medical assessment is the standard first step in treatment for eating disorders. If a child does not require urgent medical intervention, we focus on finding a therapy to help him improve his nutrition to the point where his growth and development are no longer compromised.

It's important to know that eating disorders are complex, and as doctors, we caution families against thinking that a single treatment is a magic solution. On the contrary, no single therapy can possibly provide the answer for every patient. That's why medical teams work with parents to make sure their child's treatment fits their resources and capacity, and to determine which treatment makes sense to start with, knowing that full recovery may require a sequence of treatments at different stages. Below are the most common interventions.

Psychotherapies

-> Family-based Treatment (FBT)

Ravi's doctors have recommended FBT for him and his family. FBT is the most common treatment for childhood and adolescent eating disorders because it's a flexible form of traditional family therapy that recognizes that no family is entirely the same and that parents are in the best position to help their kids.

The goal of FBT is to educate and empower parents to take charge of their child's eating through structured meal plans until her weight is restored; then the child is gradually given back control of her food intake and physical activity. During this process, a therapist supports the parents and their child, educating them about eating disorders, defusing tensions and challenges that may arise, and ensuring that the child is addressing her symptoms and working to achieve a healthy weight. Once the child is well enough, the therapy focuses on identifying and treating the underlying psychological vulnerabilities that paved the way for the eating disorder, which may mean the child participates in other therapies, such as cognitive behavior therapy for anxiety, or trauma therapy to deal with historical abuse.

While there have been some promising studies on the effectiveness of FBT for adolescents with bulimia nervosa, it has the best results when used to treat anorexia. FBT is more effective at helping children achieve and maintain a healthy weight than individual therapy with only the young patient or traditional family therapies that encourage parents to remove themselves from their child's food choices and eating, leaving the child to make his or her own decisions.[27] It's the focus on parental intervention that also makes FBT a promising treatment for younger children with ARFID, though research on successful therapies for ARFID is at a relatively early stage compared with anorexia and bulimia.

However, as with any treatment, there are limitations to FBT. Younger patients at an early stage of illness and without other mental disorders, and families who manage to keep their emotional cool during the arduous refeeding process, do best in FBT. Older, more psychiatrically unwell patients, and families with high levels of conflict—whether from exhaustion and desperation at dealing with their child's illness, or, in some cases, parents' own mental health challenges—do not do as well with this treatment and require more individualized approaches.[28]

−> Cognitive Behavior Therapy (CBT)

For older children who are not as open to their parents' involvement or for those with underlying mood and anxiety disorders, we recommend

CBT-E, an adapted form of enhanced cognitive behavior therapy, designed specifically for eating disorders.[29] As we described previously, CBT is a type of psychotherapy that helps patients look at the links between their thinking (and its distortions), feelings, and behaviors. CBT-E adds additional concrete strategies that focus on changing behaviors that have been maintaining the eating disorder. Younger children with anorexia nervosa may not respond as well to CBT because it relies on the child having some motivation. So, in situations where the child or adolescent does not wish to participate, we rely on the parent to motivate their child while we figure out how to connect with the child.

CBT has been shown to be quite effective for adolescent and adult patients with bulimia, particularly when partnered with structured eating approaches,[30] because it helps patients see the false beliefs they have about foods and their bodies, and the influence of these thoughts on their eating patterns, body image, self-esteem, and relationships. For this very reason, CBT may also prove to be instrumental in treating children with ARFID because it allows the child to understand why he or she is repulsed by certain foods and coaches parents on how to coax their child to eat.

-> Partial Hospitalization Treatment

If a child has significant medical or psychiatric symptoms and hasn't responded to initial interventions, then we recommend partial hospitalization treatment (also referred to as day hospital or day treatment programs). That way, they can be monitored more closely—both medically and psychologically—while receiving intensive treatment but remain at home with their families.

In extreme situations, where a child's weight is so low that it predisposes her to life-threatening medical complications, we have to resort to inpatient treatment, which means admitting her to the hospital for round-the-clock monitoring. Some children agree to this, but others refuse. If a child refuses and their life is in danger, most countries have laws that authorize physicians to hospitalize patients involuntarily if they are in a life-threatening medical state, irrespective of age. Some but not all jurisdictions have age-specific laws that allow parents of children under a certain age to make treatment decisions on their behalf. Once admitted, the majority of our patients—even the ones who don't want to be there—respond within a couple of days to the constant support from mental health staff and intensive treatment and are able to increase their food intake and weight, at least in the short term. In a few rare cases, patients may require nasogastric tube feedings to medically stabilize them. In these instances, a thin tube is inserted through a nostril, via the nasal passage, through the esophagus to the stomach, to deliver nutrition directly to the stomach.

These are the most common treatments for eating disorders. You'll notice that we haven't discussed medication. Treating childhood anorexia or bulimia rarely involves pharmaceuticals. As we frequently tell our patients and families, the best and most important medicine for an eating disorder is food. Children who experience crippling anxiety or depression at low weights will frequently see these improve simply with better nutrition and weight restoration. For reference, the tables at the end of the chapter review less common psychotherapies and some of the medications that are used when more established therapies are unsuccessful. When it comes to treatment, our final and most important message is that prevention—or, if already too late, early identification and treatment—are every parent's best defense against a disease that can rob children of their medical and psychological health.

After Treatment

A year after his first appointment with Dr. Monarch, Ravi is discharged from the hospital's outpatient eating disorders clinic to the care of his family physician. His weight is back up to where it was when he first started dieting, and he has grown substantially taller. He is playing hockey again but has not returned to running, telling his parents that he thinks it's safer for him to stick to sports where there is a clear start and stop time, at least for now.

He and Sanjay and Anita had some standoffs early on in treatment, usually triggered by his parents pushing him to eat more than he felt comfortable with. Ravi was convinced that he was becoming fat as a result of medically necessary weight restoration, but his parents held firm and persisted. Najma and Gaurev played essential roles in encouraging their brother, gently teasing him and their parents when mealtimes became tense, reminding Ravi of how much they wanted him to be able to join in family activities, and sometimes attending family treatment sessions.

Now, twelve months later at a final appointment, their family therapist asks Ravi what he learned from his treatment.

Ravi takes a moment to answer. "That I need to take care of my body, and feeding it properly is part of that. That I can't expect to be perfect. That my family really loves me, even when I am horrible to them."

Sanjay hands Anita a tissue so she can wipe away her tears, and he can pretend he isn't on the verge of weeping as well. They both know that Ravi still has a way to go and many challenges to face, but the last year has brought them a new, hard-won confidence in their family's strength and ability to work together to support one another.

Other Psychotherapies

Therapy	Description
Cognitive remediation therapy (CRT)	Targets rigid, inflexible thinking styles, and encourages patients to focus on the big picture, to multitask, and to be flexible rather than sticking to usual routines.[31] A more recently used type of psychotherapy for patients with anorexia nervosa.
Emotion-focused family therapy (EFFT)	Works with patients to accept and learn from their emotions. It has been adapted to augment FBT by helping parents to coach their children to express and manage emotions constructively rather than seeking to control them through eating behaviors and weight control.[32]
Acceptance and commitment therapy (ACT)	Encourages patients to accept their internal emotional states without judgement and to give up attempts to control their emotions that cause distress and tension. In addition, ACT encourages individuals to choose a treatment course based on personal values.
Dialectical behavior therapy (DBT)	Adapts Buddhist meditation, or mindfulness, to help patients accept themselves and their current circumstances, and helps them develop skills to increase their distress tolerance, find ways that are not self-destructive to manage strong emotions, and be more effective at communicating with others. A therapy for patients whose eating disorder symptoms include extreme emotional ups and downs and who struggle with self-harm impulses and suicidal thoughts and behaviors.

Medications

Medication	Description
Selective serotonin reuptake inhibitors (SSRIs)	For some children with severe anxiety or obsessive-compulsive symptoms that contribute to an eating disorder or get in the way of recovery, we prescribe SSRIs. These take longer to be effective than benzodiazepines, which are sometimes prescribed for adults to take during an anxiety attack, but are highly addictive, which is why we do not prescribe them for children and adolescents except in emergencies. SSRIs are far preferable, given that patients with eating disorders are already at a higher risk of addiction.
Antipsychotics	These are used to combat the agitation and almost delusional fear of food that can characterize severe anorexia. A small number of studies have shown that hospitalized children at very low weights respond well to very small doses. The children gained more weight more quickly than did children at comparable weights who did not take the medication. However, antipsychotics have significant side effects and can lead to adverse events. In general, it is important to seek expert advice before using any medications, as the risks often outweigh the potential rewards, though in some cases, they are worth considering.

Sleep Disorders

A Child in Distress

Javier rummages in his jacket for his cell phone and calls his ex-wife, Rita. "I can't get Camila out of bed. I've tried everything: dripping cold water on her, pulling the sheets off the bed, yelling. I feel like a monster, and none of it worked anyway. She's going to miss school again. She hasn't made it there yet for a full day this week. And I'm late for work again! I can't do this anymore."

Javier and Rita's oldest daughter, Camila, is in danger of failing twelfth grade and squandering her chance to get into the college she'd hoped to attend.

"We can't keep rescuing her, Javier," Rita says. "She's pretty much an adult, and she has to learn the hard way that only she can turn this around."

Javier would have an easier time agreeing with his ex's tough love approach if he believed Camila's inability to get out of bed in the morning was wilful. But he has seen their daughter, a conscientious and diligent student, set three different alarms at night, complete her homework, and pack her knapsack for school the night before, only to sleep through her alarms and miss another morning of classes.

The problem is that Camila always struggles to fall asleep. When she's staying with Javier, he will frequently get up to fetch his daughter an herbal tea or stroke her back until she dozes off. At his ex's, Rita leaves Camila to her own devices after eleven at night. Neither approach seems to be working; recently, Camila has withdrawn from her friends, and she stopped attending dance classes. Last week, Javier and Rita met with Camila's vice principal, Ms. Marconi, who suggested that Camila switch to online courses to allow her to complete her work on her own schedule. While Javier appreciates the administrator's flexibility, he's worried about the impact that long days alone at home, away from friends and face-to-face social contact, will have on Camila.

To make matters worse, Javier's boss told him that a continued pattern of absences would have a significant impact on his upcoming annual performance review. Javier can't afford to lose his job.

The only light at the end of the tunnel is that their family doctor offered to make an appointment for Camila with a sleep specialist. But Javier should have followed up on that weeks ago. So why didn't he? Because secretly he's afraid the specialist will tell him that Camila's problems are all his fault.

He says goodbye to Rita and climbs the stairs to Camila's room. He reminds himself that their daughter is a great kid, even if her grades are slipping and she's having some problems right now.

He walks into the bedroom. Camila is a lump tangled in covers. Javier pulls away the sheets.

"What time is it?" Camila cries, shuddering. "I'm freezing."

"Eight thirty. Come on, sweetheart. Let's try again. We're both going to be incredibly late if you don't move right now."

"I can't, Dad. Honestly, I didn't fall asleep until five. I feel sick. I need to sleep."

Javier forces himself to keep his voice even. "Camila, if you can't get to school, you'll have to switch to online courses for the rest of the year."

"I know, Dad. I know. I don't know what else to do. I'm so tired. I can't even move." Camila starts to cry. The shadows under her eyes look like old bruises, and her skin is ashen.

"You'll feel better once you get dressed and have breakfast. We can do this. Once you're at school, you usually find it easier to stay awake."

Javier stays in the room until his daughter actually climbs out of bed. Camila makes it downstairs, moving as though she is underwater. She sips at the hot sweet tea Javier has ready but turns away from the breakfast sandwich. Javier wraps it in plastic to take with them in the car. He has bigger battles than breakfast right now.

As soon as he drops off Camila at school, Javier calls their family doctor and asks him to make an appointment to see the sleep disorders specialist. They can't continue like this.

What is a sleep disorder?

After reading the above vignette, you may think that Camila is suffering from typical teenage sleep problems. And it's true that at some point every parent struggles with getting his or her child to go to sleep or wake up in the morning. These are extremely common issues in young children, and in the absence of a clear medical or psychiatric cause, they're generally considered behavioral and developmental rather than full-on disorders. This is not to say that sleep issues aren't a major source of distress for parents. Children who won't fall asleep on their own, who find any number of reasons to come into a parent's room for comfort during the night, and whose bedtime routines take up a good ninety minutes or more of parental time all cause parents stress. But in order for a child's sleep to be characterized as a disorder, there have to be daytime consequences, which include fatigue, difficulty managing their emotions and behavior, inattention, and fluctuations in mood. Javier is noticing all of these with Camila.

So what exactly is a sleep disorder? A sleep disorder is when problems with the quantity, quality, and timing of an individual's sleep cause difficulties in her day-to-day functioning and cause her distress. During sleep, we alternate between two different kinds of sleep, starting with non-rapid eye movement (NREM) sleep, then rapid eye movement (REM) sleep, and then back to NREM, then REM, and on and on. NREM constitutes about 70 percent to 80 percent of our sleep. Each cycle of NREM sleep has three separate stages, ranging from superficial to deep sleep. Deep sleep is what we need to feel rested when we wake up. REM fills the remainder of our sleep and is responsible for most of our dreaming. Over the course of the night, the time we spend in REM increases, with its longest periods happening in the last third. In sleep disorders, this entire sleep pattern is disrupted. For example, when those suffering from narcolepsy—a sleep disorder characterized by intense daytime drowsiness and sudden sleep attacks—fall asleep, they experience REM before NREM, instead of the other way around.[1]

While sleep disorders may seem like a minor mental health issue, when left untreated, poor sleep can contribute to a number of negative outcomes for children and adolescents, including poor growth, erratic appetite, weight gain, decreased school and work performance, increased risk of drowsiness while driving, behavioral changes, inattention, changes in mood, and anxiety symptoms. A sleep disorder may also be a sign of another psychiatric disorder, such as ADHD, autism spectrum disorder, or mood and anxiety disorders, which is why if you're concerned your child is suffering from a sleep disorder, have him assessed by his doctor.

What are the different types of sleep disorders and their warning signs?

Insomnia

Behavioral insomnia is the best-known childhood sleep disorder, affecting approximately 25 percent of boys and girls.[2] Symptoms include difficulty falling and staying asleep and waking up exceptionally early in the morning, all of which leave the sufferer feeling tired the next day. When these symptoms continue and begin to impair the child's day-to-day life, these sleep disturbances are diagnosed as insomnia.[3] In younger children, insomnia can mask separation anxiety or bedtime fears where the real issue is the child's discomfort at being away from parents and/or being in a dark room alone. In older children, insomnia is more likely caused by the use of screens at bedtime and during the night. It's particularly common for teens with an underlying anxiety or mood disorder to experience delays in falling asleep.

Nightmares

Nightmares are a common form of sleep disturbance that tends to affect girls more than boys.[4] These are distressing and frightening dreams that occur during REM sleep and may wake the child during the night or be upsetting to recall the next day. Nightmares constitute a disorder only if they are frequent and severe enough to interfere consistently with a child getting sufficient sleep. By themselves, nightmares are not signs of anxiety, hidden trauma, or unhappiness, although a recurring nightmare focused on similar themes may point to a specific cause.

Parasomnias

Parasomnias—sleep talking, sleep terrors, sleepwalking—are different from nightmares in that the child remains asleep despite the disruption of screaming, moving, and sometimes aggression, and the child rarely remembers what happened the next day. Parasomnias are more common in boys than in girls, and they run in families. Sleep terrors appear most often in preschool-age children, while sleepwalking appears predominantly in children between ages six and twelve years, but both rarely persist into adolescence.

Sleepwalking can be concerning because it places a child at risk if he or she attempts to navigate stairs or leave the house while asleep. Parents can ensure their child's safety by removing potential obstacles from his immediate sleep vicinity and by installing safety gates so that a child cannot exit the home. Still, the major consequence of sleepwalking is the disruption to the child's period of restorative sleep, which leads to feeling fatigued the next day. If parents can gently guide their child back to bed without waking him or her, this disturbance can be mitigated. In our experience, parasomnias end up impacting parents' sleep more than the child's.

Sleep-Disordered Breathing

Sleep-disordered breathing, or obstructive sleep apnea (OSA), is relatively common in young children and is usually due to a developmental delay in their tonsils and adenoids in relation to their upper airways. As a result, their airway constricts or collapses intermittently overnight, causing abnormal pauses in breathing known as apneas.[5] Both tonsils and adenoids, which are clumps of lymphatic tissue situated at the back of the throat and nasal cavity, respectively, protect against infection and begin to shrink during adolescence and often disappear by adulthood. More recently, we have learned that obesity can contribute to OSA because there is additional pressure on a child's upper airway. Symptoms of OSA include persistent snoring, frequent awakenings, and insufficient REM sleep.

Circadian Rhythm Sleep-Wake Disorders

This sleep disorder occurs when two of the bodily systems that regulate sleep are out of sync and thus unable to function. The first body system is the circadian rhythm cycle, a twenty-four-hour cycle that regulates the body's biological clock and is affected by environmental triggers such as light and darkness. When a sleeping person is exposed to light, the retinal cells in the back of their eyes send a signal to the brain that it's daytime and therefore time to wake. The second body system is the sleep-wake system, which works with the circadian rhythm cycle to track the amount of sleep we get; it's like a virtual "spring" in our brains that winds up tighter the longer we are awake until the pressure is so great that we fall asleep.

When these systems aren't working, the body cannot fall asleep until well into the early morning hours and cannot wake up until the afternoon. This is known as delayed sleep phase disorder (DSPD), a condition that affects up to 16 percent of adolescents. One in ten referrals among all age groups to sleep clinics for chronic insomnia are related to DSPD.

These are the most common and persistent sleep disorders. At the end of the chapter, we've included a table outlining other sleep disorders and their symptoms.

What are the risk factors for developing a sleep disorder?

Environmental Factors

Here's some inspiring news: parents set the stage for healthy sleep behaviors and can encourage good habits, which we'll discuss in a moment. While it's not unusual for a child to struggle with going to bed, how parents respond is key. Teaching children to fall asleep alone and self-soothe if they wake up (when you and their health care provider feel they are ready to do so) ensures that both you and your child are getting enough sleep. Even if a child is suffering from parasomnias, it's important to establish boundaries so that when the child outgrows the parasomnia (as most children do), he has a routine to fall back on. That said, environment is only one part of the puzzle, and often there is a contributing biological or psychological reason for a child to develop a sleep disorder.

Parents will be all too familiar with another environmental factor that contributes to our children's sleep problems: technology. For instance, the blue light emitted by cell phones suppresses the hormone melatonin,[6] which is secreted overnight by the pineal gland in the brain and plays an important role in our natural sleep-wake cycle. Another contributing factor: the mental stimulation from, say, scrolling social media on phones and other electronic devices also keeps children and adolescents from the sleep they desperately need.[7]

Biological Factors

Certain sleep disorders are more common in family members, including restless legs syndrome (RLS) and narcolepsy, both explained at chapter's end.[8] But the most common biological risk factor is the enlarged tonsils and adenoids associated with sleep apnea.

Some medications, too, can disrupt sleep, such as stimulants used to treat ADHD; asthma medications, which can cause excitability; nonprescription cold and cough medications containing pseudoephedrine and caffeine; corticosteroid medications (which decrease inflammation and reduce the activity of the immune system); and certain antidepressants. Nicotine, marijuana, and other recreational drugs can also contribute to sleep disturbance in adolescents.

Psychological Factors

Sleep disorders often occur in the context of other psychiatric disorders, including mood or anxiety disorders, autism, and ADHD. Children with these conditions often struggle with going to bed at a regular time, falling asleep, staying asleep during the night, waking up in the morning, and daytime sleepiness.[9] To complicate matters further, medications employed in managing these disorders are known to contribute to sleep problems, particularly insomnia. Typically, the worse the sleep disturbance, the worse the symptoms of the other disorder.

What can parents do to help prevent sleep disorders?

There are effective preventative strategies that parents can employ almost as soon as their child is ready for his or her own bed. Below we've listed the most important ways to promote healthy sleep practices in your home. Incorporating these steps early with young children will go a long way in preventing sleep problems.

- Keep the sleeping area dark and peaceful.
- Ensure a comfortably cool room temperature.
- Make your child go to bed and wake up at the same time, even on weekends.
- Have a consistent bedtime routine: consider a warm shower or bath, relaxation exercises, meditation, and herbal tea.
- Keep your child's bed for sleep. If he cannot fall asleep, get him out of bed to do something else relaxing before trying again.
- Electronic entertainment should be off-limits for at least an hour before bedtime, preferably more. This includes phones, televisions, computers, and so on. Keep these devices outside the sleeping area.
- For children over five, avoid napping during the day.

- Discourage your child from exercising in the hours before bedtime; instead, encourage him or her to engage in vigorous physical activity earlier in the day.
- Expose your child to natural light as much as possible during the day and especially in the morning; this helps regulate his or her circadian and sleep-wake systems.
- Make sure your child isn't hungry before he goes to bed, but avoid serving a large meal late in the evening.
- Keep your son or daughter away from caffeinated food or beverages, including kid favorites Coca-Cola and chocolate, or other stimulants in the late afternoon and evening.

For young children who don't have any particular psychiatric or medical disorder but have never developed good sleep habits and have difficulty falling and staying asleep at night, it's important to teach them to fall asleep on their own. Parents have told us that they are concerned about intervening in their children's bedtime routine, fearing that it will exacerbate stress or behavioral or emotional problems, or negatively impact the parent-child relationship. We suggest something called "gradual extinction." Research shows that this technique has positive outcomes and assuages the above concerns that may cause parents to hesitate before intervening.[10] Here's how it works:

If your child cries once she is left alone to fall asleep, encourage her to self-soothe by waiting a few minutes before responding. If she continues to cry, leave her alone for increasingly longer durations of time; or stay with her at bedtime but gradually move away from the bed until she can fall asleep without a parent present in the room.

For parents who wish to learn more about behavioral interventions that are associated with earlier and improved sleep patterns in children, we have included some further reading material in the resources section at the end of the book.

Reaching a Diagnosis

Six weeks later, Javier and Camila are due to meet Dr. Neil Stein, a child and adolescent psychiatrist specializing in sleep disorders. Prior to the appointment, the teenager's family doctor examined her and tested her blood to rule out medical causes for her sleep problems, such as asthma, gastroesophageal reflux, thyroid disease, low iron, and allergies, among others. Javier, Rita, and Camila also completed lengthy questionnaires about Camila's sleep history and habits, and Camila has been keeping a sleep diary. All of this information was sent to Dr. Stein in advance of their consultation.

Dr. Stein, a tall, kind-faced man in his forties, comes out to the reception area to greet them. He asks Camila if she would like to meet with him alone or include Javier for part of the appointment.

"I'd like my father to come."

Javier is touched by Camila's willingness to include him. Maybe he hasn't made as much of a mess trying to help his daughter as he thinks?

Once in his office, Dr. Stein turns to Camila. "What made you decide to seek more help?" he asks.

Camila tells him that her sleep problems have taken over her life. "I agreed to come to the appointment because I'm hoping there is a medication I can take. My family doctor wasn't comfortable prescribing anything."

Javier draws an audible breath. Camila hadn't told him this before. Recently, he discovered that his own mother, Sofia, had become physically dependent upon Valium to sleep and needed to be weaned off.

Javier has no intention of letting his seventeen-year-old daughter become similarly dependent.

"We generally don't look to medications until we have exhausted other effective strategies," the physician tells her, "given that medications tend to only help in the short term and can cause a host of other problems, but we can certainly discuss them as part of an overall treatment approach."

Dr. Stein's calm, measured answer allays Javier's fears.

"I have your questionnaires and the sleep diary here, but could you tell me a bit more about when these sleep problems began?"

Taking turns, Javier and Camila explain that Camila has always struggled with sleep. As an infant, she rarely slept through the night. At age three, she started sleepwalking and suffered from sleep terrors. Javier used to invite her to sleep with him and Rita, just to ease their daughter's fear. What Javier doesn't say is that his then wife often disagreed with this practice, but cosleeping in Javier's parents' culture was quite common. This was one of many reasons he and Rita grew apart and divorced.

Although Camila eventually grew out of night terrors, she never managed to establish a predictable or restful sleep pattern. Then, last summer, Camila got a job at a local movie theater, which meant she rarely returned home before one or two in the morning. She would sleep late into the afternoon before heading in for an evening shift at five. Although she and Javier talked about getting back into a sleep schedule more conducive to school, this never happened. Now, in twelfth grade, Camila routinely stays awake until three or four in the morning on her computer doing homework and posting on social media, which is why she struggles every morning to wake up.

Dr. Stein makes notes throughout, and when they're finished, he smiles at them. "The good news is that nothing concerning has shown up on Camila's physical exam or blood work. At this point, I'd like to hear the rest of the story from Camila on her own."

Javier wants to protest but instead politely excuses himself from the room. About forty minutes later, Dr. Stein invites Javier back into his office.

"I'm reasonably convinced that the two of you identified the main causes of Camila's sleep problems when you explained the impact of her summer job schedule and now her academic stress and anxiety. But given her long history of issues with sleep, I'm recommending that Camila undergo a sleep study where she stays overnight at a sleep laboratory."

"Will I be hooked up to a bunch of machines?" Camila asks. "I've seen that on TV."

Dr. Stein chuckles. "Yes, it's a lot like that." He explains that they'll measure her brain wave activity, muscle and eye movements, and heart rhythm. "This gives us a picture of how long it takes you to fall asleep, how long you stay asleep, and the ratio of time you spend asleep versus awake.[11] Don't worry. We're going to find out what's going on and get you the help you need."

Javier squeezes Camila's hand. That's all he wants.

A month later, they're back in Dr. Stein's office, looking with bemusement at the graphic results of the sleep study: a long ticker tape of squiggles. In the intervening weeks, Camila has dutifully followed the doctor's recommendations to improve her sleep, including moving her phone, laptop, and television out of her room at night. Although her sleep is not much better, she has made it to school on time more often.

Dr. Stein spreads out the tape in front of them. "This is like learning a foreign language. First the good news. There's no evidence here of sleep apnea or a pattern consistent with narcolepsy. We're also not seeing restless legs syndrome or any of the other sleep issues that are more challenging to treat."

Javier breathes a sigh of relief.

"What we are seeing is called a circadian rhythm sleep-wake disorder, with the name delayed sleep phase type. It's very common in adolescents."

"Will it go away?" Camila asks, her voice tremulous.

"Yes. It is very treatable. In everyday terms, what it means is exactly what the two of you already know: Camila, your body cannot fall asleep at the time that we would expect it to, and instead it falls asleep just as most people are waking. This is why you can't get up in the morning and sleep most of the day. Now, if you were working a night shift, this might be fine, but for a teenager who needs to get to school, get homework done, have the energy to see friends, and do all the other things you want to do outside school, it's a disaster."

"What caused it?" Javier asks, fearing that his permissive parenting regarding sleep will be the answer.

"It's hard to know. Many teenagers have this type of sleep disorder, and often there are many causes. Camila's early sleeping problems likely put her at higher risk for developing a sleep disorder later in adolescence. The change in sleep routine at your job last summer was probably a major contributor. And Camila, you told me at your first appointment that you tend to worry and ruminate late at night and then use electronic screens to distract yourself, all of which exacerbates existing problems and leads to a sleep disorder."

Anxious thoughts? Javier thinks to himself. He didn't know about that part, but he's grateful Camila shared that with Dr. Stein.

The psychiatrist continues. "I am confident we can help you with a combination of what we call sleep hygiene strategies and therapy."

Camila grimaces. "What about medication? You said at the first appointment we could talk about it. One of my friends is taking melatonin, and another is on something called Ativan."

Javier bites his tongue. Dr. Stein looks thoughtful. "Are either of them finding these helpful?" he asks.

"My friend says the Ativan helped at the beginning but not now. My friend who takes the melatonin says sometimes yes, sometimes no."

"We wouldn't generally recommend Ativan. It's a benzodiazepine, and those are all addictive. They have significant effects on your thinking and short-term memory, which are obviously essential for students. They also don't work in the long term."

"What about melatonin?" Camila persists.

"It can be helpful for people with jet lag or with children who have a developmental disorder, but beyond that, we don't have a lot of evidence to suggest that it's worth taking. Because it is not a prescription medication, there's no quality control, which means you cannot be entirely sure what you are getting. More important, the vast majority of sleep disorders of the type you are experiencing respond very well to cognitive behavioral therapy and improved sleep practices, without the need of any additional medication."

"Okay," Camila says. "Let's give the therapy a shot."

As Dr. Stein ushers them both out of the office, Javier feels as though a heavy weight has been lifted from his shoulders. His daughter's sleep problems are real, they have a name, and they can be treated—without a potentially dangerous medication. He senses the path ahead will not be easy, but he can imagine a day in the future when Camila's life might not be upended by her sleep disorder.

What are the treatments for sleep disorders?

As we saw above, the first step in treatment is to make behavioral changes; then therapy is recommended as needed, with medication tapped as a last resort. Below we've outlined a bit more about each of these treatments so that if your child is diagnosed with a sleep disorder, you'll have an initial sense of the options available.

Behavioral Interventions

Behavioral changes are the most effective way to develop good sleep hygiene: a set of practices that promote better sleep. We described many of them in our earlier section on preventative strategies for sleep disorders.

For children with parasomnias, safety proofing the home is essential, as is reducing anxiety and stress by whatever means available. For example, ensuring that your child has lots of physical activity earlier in the day can help reduce anxiety. There are also relaxation apps that children can listen to before going to bed, ranging from the sound of waves to guided meditations to new age music. And, of course, we recommend the tried-and-true tradition of reading to your child before bed. With the help of smart phones and home video cameras, parents can also figure out when their child's parasomnia is likely to occur and wake him or her up before it starts.[12]

Psychotherapies

CBT-i, a type of cognitive behavior therapy specifically adapted for insomnia, is extremely effective. Using cognitive therapy techniques to help patients identify distorted and irrational thoughts and beliefs, CBT-i reduces the anxiety and arousal that trying to fall asleep evokes in people with insomnia.[13] CBT-i also uses mindfulness meditation and relaxation techniques to help children learn to regulate their emotions and to respond to their insomnia with an appropriate range of feelings.

Medical/Surgical Interventions

For children whose sleep disorders are related to breathing problems, treatment may involve surgically removing enlarged tonsils and adenoids or the use of a continuous positive airway pressure (CPAP) machine, a face mask worn at night to keep the child's airway open. His doctor will also look at addressing any relevant allergies and environmental irritants. And, of course, if obesity is the cause, treatment will include exercise and a food plan designed around healthy eating, drawing on all food groups rather than severe calorie restriction to help the child achieve a healthier weight.[14]

Medications

As Dr. Stein told Camila and Javier, medications are rarely used for sleep disorders, only when other interventions are not successful alone or when the child suffers from another psychiatric condition—and even then, they're prescribed carefully and sparingly. Before adding medications, the first step is to explore whether a child is on a medication for another medical or psychiatric condition that may be inadvertently contributing to the sleep disorder and adjusting or discontinuing that medication if appropriate.

Diphenhydramine (Benadryl) and dimenhydrinate (Gravol, Dramamine) are two of the most commonly used over-the-counter medications by parents to help children sleep. While they are generally thought by parents to be benign, both can cause unsteadiness and impair learning.[15] There are reports of seizures in infants, and, at high doses in older children, agitation, nightmares, irritability, and even psychotic symptoms. Teenagers can also misuse dimenhydrinate to get high. For these reasons, we don't recommend their use.

Like Dr. Stein, we discourage the use of benzodiazepines such as Ativan and Valium, as the risk of developing an addiction and the negative impact on cognitive functioning are just too great. Initial doses of these medications have a short-lived effect, with users becoming tolerant and thus requiring higher and higher doses. In some cases, sleep disturbance worsens after discontinuing use.

Melatonin is probably the most widely used over-the-counter sleep

aid. While there is some scientific evidence that it is effective in helping children with autism, ADHD, and intellectual disabilities fall asleep
more quickly and stay asleep, we don't have research yet to show that it is
useful as a sleep aid in children with sleep disturbance who are otherwise
healthy.[16] Also, as Dr. Stein alluded to, melatonin is not a regulated substance, which raises concern about its quality control and safety.

There are other medications that we haven't mentioned here, but as
with any prescriptions, it's important to talk to your child's doctor about
any potential downsides. Again, medications for sleep disorders are typically used only after behavioral interventions and other therapies have
been exhausted. When they are ordered, it's only for a week or two at a
time to try to reestablish a more regular sleep rhythm.

After Treatment

The first month of Dr. Stein's prescribed treatment is grim, primarily
because of the severe adjustments to Camila's habits that Javier must
enforce. On her new schedule, the seventeen-year-old gets up at six
o'clock—which gives Javier a full hour to get his daughter moving before
he has to get ready for work. Dr. Stein told Camila she can sleep in one
hour longer on the weekend. Before supper, Camila takes an hourlong
walk, rain or shine, and goes to bed at ten o'clock. Javier makes sure to
confiscate all of her electronics two hours before bedtime. Camila pro-
tests that she's still awake half the night, but her grey skin and the dark
circles under her eyes strengthen Javier's resolve every morning. For the
first three weeks, Camila decided to stay solely at Javier's, but then she
returned to Rita's apartment for the weekend and reported back that
she had been able to stick to her routine and managed to sleep about six
hours each night.

The next month is a bit better. Camila still complains of sleepless nights but looks less tired and seems more engaged with her schoolwork and dance classes, which she has resumed. She attends the CBT-i mindfulness group regularly, where she has learned to meditate. She finds it helpful in many aspects of her life, not just sleep. She has more of an appetite, and the color in her face has improved.

By the third month, Camila tells Javier that most nights she sleeps right through. On the few nights when she wakes, she reminds herself not to worry, practices her meditations, and falls back asleep within an hour. She has decided to drop two classes and take an extra year of high school so she can have a late start in the mornings, but her grades are up to where they were before. Overall, both Javier and Rita see a significant change in their daughter. She's more cheerful, focused, and energetic.

On a Sunday evening when Rita drops off Camila after a weekend away at Rita's parents' summer cabin, she gives Javier a hug. "You cracked it. And without making her feel we're the enemy. Well done. I'm really grateful. You were right, and I was wrong."

Javier can feel his face flush. "Now, if only we could have said that a few more times ten years ago, who knows where we'd be now?"

The two parents hug as Camila squeezes around them with her bag. "Come on, Dad, I need to eat and then finish my homework. I want to get to bed early because I have tryouts for the dance troupe tomorrow morning."

Her words are music to both her parents' ears.

Other Sleep Disorders

Disorder	Description
Enuresis	A sleep disorder characterized by bed wetting. Now, most young children struggle with bladder control at some point in their development, but when frequent bed-wetting episodes disturb their sleep, we call this a disorder. Bed wetting is more common in boys, occurring in 10% to 15% of five-year-olds and 6% to 8% of eight-year-olds. The good news is that enuresis declines to 1% to 2% by fifteen years of age.
Bruxism	The involuntary grinding of one's teeth and/or jaw while asleep. It can affect sleep quality and, in some rare cases, result in dental damage. Insomnia can lead to increased bruxism and vice versa. Dental devices such as mouth guards and relaxation strategies are common treatment interventions.
Hypersomnolence	Excessive daytime sleepiness caused most often by poor or inadequate sleep at night, but it can also result from some mood disorders and medical conditions.
Narcolepsy	A rare sleep disorder characterized by excessive daytime sleepiness. Symptoms can include cataplexy (sudden, involuntary muscle weakness that can cause the person to collapse, usually triggered by strong emotion) and sleep paralysis (a temporary inability to move that usually occurs when falling asleep or waking). It is the only sleep disorder to warrant medication as the primary and only curative treatment.

Disorder	Description
Restless legs syndrome (RLS) and periodic limb movement disorder (PLMD)	Related sleep disorders characterized by an uncomfortable and persistent need to move one's lower limbs. While RLS and PLMD can occur after long periods of inactivity, they most often come on at bedtime, which leads to difficulty falling asleep and frequent wakening.[17, 18] Their cause is unknown, although they may have a genetic component, and have been associated with low iron, diabetes, and certain neurological illnesses.

Depression, Trauma, and Suicidal Thoughts

A Child in Distress

It's four in the morning, and Sara is in the emergency department in her nightgown, winter boots, and down coat. Down the hall, her sixteen-year-old daughter, Chana, is being treated for a drug overdose. An hour earlier, Sara had woken up for no reason, her heart racing, and felt compelled to check on her daughter—something she hasn't done in years. She found Chana unconscious on her bedroom floor with an empty bottle of Tylenol next to her. Sara opened her mouth to scream—she doesn't remember if she produced any sound—and reached for the phone to call 911.

Now her mind is percolating with questions. Why would her daughter take those pills? Had she really intended to kill herself? Chana has been more withdrawn in recent months, and her grades have slipped, which has never happened before. Sara has also noticed abrasions on Chana's thighs that haven't seemed to heal, but when she asked about them, her daughter claimed they were from soccer practice, and Sara didn't pursue it. She wondered briefly if Chana was cutting herself, but felt certain that if anything major was happening in her teenager's life, Chana would talk to her. They have always been open with each other, although now Sara realizes her confidence has been misplaced. If only her husband, Max, were still alive, he would know what to do. But he died six years ago, and she is on her own with this. She cannot lose Chana, too.

Sara is still searching her memory for missed clues or hints when a young woman enters the family lounge and introduces herself as Dr. Cadence Adebeyo, the emergency medicine physician. She ushers Sara into a small, empty, windowless room occupied by a stretcher, two chairs, and some medical equipment.

"How is Chana? Will she be okay?" Sara asks as the physician draws the sliding door closed.

"She's okay," Dr. Adebeyo says, and Sara lets out the breath she was holding. "We've stabilized her blood pressure and heart rate, and we have pumped her stomach and started an antidote to the Tylenol she took." Her voice is calm as she walks Sara through what they know. "Her drug screen suggests she may have also taken an antidepressant: bupropion. Was Chana on any medications? Or is someone else in the house taking it?"

Sara feels as though she may vomit. "I am. I've been on it since my husband died. Chana knows I take it—I don't believe in keeping secrets from my kids—but I didn't think she knew where I kept it."

"We are reasonably confident that we intervened quickly enough to prevent Chana from having significant liver damage from the acetaminophen, and we are watching for seizures, which can sometimes occur with overdoses of bupropion. We'll have to wait and see to be certain. We are sending her up to the intensive care unit team, where they can support her breathing and her heart, and monitor her closely. Once she's settled, you are very welcome to go and sit with her."

"Thank you." All Sara wants is to see her daughter.

"You must have many questions." Dr. Adebeyo's eyes are full of concern. "Right now we're focusing on making sure Chana is okay physically. Once we know she is stable, we can change our focus to understanding what's been going on with her. The psychiatry resident who is on call overnight would like to talk with you to get some background history. Would that be okay?"

Sara nods mutely, dreading how she must seem to the staff here—disheveled, exhausted, terrified. Does she look like an incompetent mother who had no idea about her child's desperation?

Thirty minutes later, a slight man about half Sara's age introduces himself as Dr. Devin Senasinghe, the psychiatry resident on call.

"I know what you are going to ask me," Sara says. "But I honestly have no idea why this happened."

Dr. Senasinghe's face is serious yet kind. "Many parents say the same thing. Children frequently don't share suicidal thoughts with parents—for all sorts of reasons. And in our experience, parents blame themselves, although it's not something one has control over."

As he speaks, Sara's eyes fill with tears. She was expecting judgment, not understanding.

He hands her a box of tissues. "Do you feel okay to talk? May I ask you about Chana?"

"Yes," Sara replies.

"Has she ever done anything like this before?"

"No, never."

"Have you noticed any changes in Chana's behavior recently? Any stresses in her life?"

Sara tells Dr. Senasinghe that Chana has seemed different in recent months, since starting back at school in September. "She's withdrawn from her friends, her brother, and me, and her grades are the lowest they've ever been. Her appetite has been off, too, and she's complained about not sleeping at night. Lately, she's been avoiding my hugs. I thought it was just the regular moodiness that teenage girls have. In hindsight, I also think she may have been cutting herself. I can't believe what an idiot I've been."

"It's often hard for a parent to know if a change in a teenager's behavior is outside the realm of normal for their age, particularly if the teenager won't communicate. And there are many, many factors that go into an adolescent making a suicide attempt; you are not to blame for what has happened." Dr. Senasinghe's face conveys empathy that Sara senses is genuine. "Has Chana been seeing a therapist or a psychiatrist? Was she on any medication? Has there been concern about Chana using drugs?"

As Sara shakes her head to all these questions, she continues to berate herself despite the resident's reassurances. Why hadn't she worried more? Insisted Chana talk to someone? Searched her room? Pushed her more about her cuts? Isn't that what a decent parent does? Isn't that what Max would have done? The pain of not having him there at this moment is overwhelming. It's so unfair that she has to cope with this without him.

Dr. Senasinghe's voice brings Sara back to the present. "It's too early to say for sure, and there are many other possibilities to explore, but from what you're describing, it sounds like Chana may be struggling with depression."

Sara looks at him in disbelief. "Depression? Chana's always been the rock in our family; she's incredibly mature and thoughtful. Her brother, Dror, has been much more up and down. He's the one I've been worried about. In a way, Chana's taken care of both of us since my husband's death. This feels like I'll wake up, and it will turn out to be a bad dream."

"A child's suicide attempt is one of the worst things a parent has to endure. I'm sorry you are facing this. But Chana's alive, and we have an opportunity to help her." Both Dr. Senasinghe and Sara are silent for a moment before he continues. "I am going to ask the social worker on our team to check in with you tomorrow to see what you and Dror may need in the way of support. This is a terrible shock, and it's normal to feel uncertain about a lot of things."

"Thank you for being so kind. I feel such a failure to have missed this."

Dr. Senasinghe holds her gaze. "This is not about failure. And you and Chana and Dror have another chance."

As the resident walks out of the room, Sara twists the wedding ring she has worn on her right hand since Max's death. Under her breath, she asks for Max's help.

As parents, we know firsthand that the above vignette is not easy to read. But as psychiatrists, we can't stress enough how important it is for parents to understand that children and adolescents with depression, bipolar disorder, and other psychiatric disorders are at exceptionally high risk of suicidal thoughts and attempts. Suicide is the second leading cause of death among children, adolescents, and young adults between the ages of fifteen and twenty-four years old.[1] Recent US studies point to increased suicide rates over the past two decades for young people between fifteen and twenty-four, with 2017 rates at the highest point since 2000.[2] Other studies over the same period have shown an exponential rise in emergency room visits by children and adolescents presenting with suicidal thoughts or having made attempts, a rise that is consistent with what we have seen at our own hospital. While it is possible that an increased willingness to seek help and to report deaths by suicide contribute partly to this increase, there's no softening those statistics. Our hope is that we can offer you knowledge and skills so you are aware of any warning signs that your child may be experiencing suicidal thoughts and feelings and you can intervene at the earliest possible opportunity to get him or her the necessary help.

The majority of children and adolescents who think about and attempt suicide have previously received a psychiatric diagnosis—such as substance use disorder or eating disorder—but mood disorders[3, 4, 5, 6, 7] are the most common. Completed suicides have been linked, in particular, to diagnoses of bipolar disorder.[8, 9] For that reason, we are going to take some time now to explain what mood disorders are.

What is a mood disorder?

A mood disorder is a mental illness that causes an individual to experience distinct periods of altered emotions, thinking, and bodily functions (sleep, appetite, and energy). These episodes affect the person's outlook on themselves, their relationships, school and work, and the larger world. A mood disorder episode generally lasts for a finite period of time, but mood disorders are rarely limited to a single episode; in other words, people with mood disorders often experience recurrences over their lifetime. While it is common for most of us to have transient mood changes, if these changes persist beyond a couple of weeks and interfere with one's ability to function at home, at school, or with friends, it's important to consider the possibility of a mood disorder and to seek help.

What are the different types of mood disorders and their warning signs?

Depression

Most parents have heard of—and in some cases experienced—depression. It is a term often used colloquially to describe feeling sad, but speaking medically, it means more than that. Almost everyone will have periods of sadness after a hurt, loss, or disappointment, but those who also feel sluggish, apathetic, and unmotivated, and have trouble eating and sleeping (either too much or too little), may be experiencing a bout of clinical depression. They may feel numb and irritable, and not be interested in or able to experience pleasure in things that they used to enjoy. Some individuals experience both physical and psychological agitation, finding it hard to be still or to stop ruminating; others feel slowed and weighed down. Over time, their thinking becomes distorted, and they come to see themselves, their impact on other people, and their futures negatively. This progression signals that an episode of sadness has developed from an understandable response to life stresses, to a serious diagnosis of depression. People with depression may come to think of death as an escape—from their exhaustion, their sense of uselessness and guilt, and their belief they are a burden on others—which is why sufferers are at significantly higher risk for death by suicide than their healthy relatives, colleagues, and friends.

In some severe cases, depression can be accompanied by psychotic symptoms that generally reflect an individual's mood state: delusions (irrational, false beliefs) and hallucinations, where the person sees, hears, smells, tastes, or feels stimuli that don't exist. For example, a popular adolescent who has many friends, when depressed, may start to believe—without any factual evidence—that these same friends have turned on her, are talking about her unkindly, and posting false statements about her online. She may have experiences where she believes she hears her friends speaking about her negatively—when in reality there is no one around—or starts to think that complete strangers are involved in a larger conspiracy and have heard untrue and destructive rumors about her.

Up to 13 percent of North American adolescents experience major depression in a given year, with the rate in teenage girls reaching 20 percent.[10] Up to 2 percent of children experience depression before age thirteen, so it's important that parents learn to recognize the warning signs of depression, which look different in children and teens from adults.[11]

In children and teens, depression symptoms may manifest as frequent stomachaches and headaches; significant changes to sleep, appetite, and energy levels; fatigue; trouble focusing; irritability; and withdrawal from friends, family, school, and activities that the child used to enjoy. These symptoms can lead to underperforming at school. While it's typical for a teenager to experience moodiness, if he's suffering from depression, he may seem angry and irritable rather than sad, and his moods may be more reactive. For example, he may seem cheerful for limited periods with friends but at home appear sullen and unapproachable.[12] It's easy to write this off as wilful teenage rebellion, but we caution parents to look deeper into the reasons for such reactivity. Adolescents also may misuse substances, such as alcohol or drugs, in an unintended effort to self-medicate a depressive disorder. Of course, as we have pointed out in our chapter on substance use disorders, substance misuse itself can bring about depressive symptoms.

In addition to the above warning signs, there are other even more serious behaviors to look out for, including self-harm, where, like Chana, a child cuts or burns herself. Not all children who self-harm experience suicidal thoughts or behavior, and they often describe their actions as an outlet for releasing unbearable tension. However, self-harm and suicidal behavior exist on a continuum, and children who engage in self-harm are at a higher risk for attempting suicide later on, particularly when they are also struggling with mood disorders.[13, 14]

If you notice your child or adolescent hurting herself, talking about being a burden or a failure, or expressing feelings of hopelessness about the future, get her assessed by a health care professional right away. Don't simply write this off as a phase or assume these behaviors are manageable and let time go by.[15]

Bipolar Spectrum Disorders

While people with depression rarely feel happiness during their episodes of illness, individuals with bipolar disorder can have significant mood swings and go from extremes of euphoria to the depths of sadness consistent with depression within weeks or even days. These elevated, "high" moods are called either manic or hypomanic episodes. Both hypomanic and manic episodes are uncharacteristic changes in a person's mood, behavior, sense of self, and level of functioning, and may include several of the following: an inflated sense of the person's worth and abilities; heightened energy, activity, and talkativeness; an increase in unwise and risk-taking behaviors; significantly decreased need for sleep; racing thoughts; and increased distractibility. Hypomania lasts for a minimum of four days and mania, seven, with symptoms present for most of the day in both cases.

The difference between mania and hypomania lies in the severity of the symptoms and their impact on the person's life. While the changes in attitude and behavior associated with hypomania can sometimes make functioning in social settings and school or the workplace a challenge, hypomania is not associated with the level of self-destructive behavior or adverse outcomes that characterize full-blown mania. Unlike hypomania, mania can also develop into psychosis and require hospitalization to prevent the sufferer from endangering himself or others. Bipolar I disorder, by definition, includes at least one episode of mania in addition to depression and can include episodes of hypomania; bipolar II disorder refers to at least one episode of hypomania in addition to depression but never includes full-blown manic episodes. There are other variations of bipolar spectrum disorders; a table at the end of the chapter provides a full breakdown of the subtypes and their symptoms.

How can you know if your child is struggling with bipolar disorder? As parents, we know that teens tend to take more risks as they get older, but from our clinical work with parents, we also realize that there may be other challenges to figuring out if your child is experiencing hypomania or mania. For example, an adolescent experiencing hypomania may simply appear to be more self-confident, energetic, and productive than usual. Indeed, individuals with bipolar II frequently describe hypomania as seductive and enjoyable—at least until they understand that it will inevitably herald a crash into depression. A child who has appeared to recover from a significant episode of depression may actually be experiencing hypomania, but sometimes, in the absence of a diagnosis of bipolar II disorder, parents misinterpret their child's hypomanic symptoms as a return to normal. As a result of their relief at seeing their child free of depression, they see hypomania through rose-colored glasses, not the reality that this is a version of their child that they have never seen before, which can lead to a delay in treatment.

If warning signs—uncharacteristic changes in mood, energy levels, sleep patterns, and so forth—are present, parents need to talk to their children and find out more about what is contributing to any change. Specific examples of unusual behavior such as running away, staying out all night, shoplifting, joyriding, drug taking, and high-risk sexual behaviors from an adolescent who has never exhibited these types of behaviors before are all indicators that something may be wrong.

What are the risk factors for developing a mood disorder and suicidal thoughts and behaviors?

No single factor causes a child to develop a mood disorder and suicidal thoughts and behaviors; it's usually a mix of environmental, biological, and psychological risk factors. The higher the number of risk factors, the higher an individual child's risk, but do keep in mind that risk factors do not make a diagnosis—they are only markers of vulnerability.

Environmental Factors

The environmental causes of mood disorders are many and often overlapping: bullying, family and parental marital conflict, academic failures, relationship breakups, and social isolation have all been identified as contributors.[16] Certain groups of children and adolescents are particularly predisposed, including gay, bisexual, and gender-diverse children, who are all at much greater risk of mood disorders,[17, 18] self-harm, and suicide attempts,[19] particularly if they are not supported by their families.[20] LGBTQ2S youth frequently live in environments characterized by stigma, discrimination, and bullying, all of which are known to raise mental health risks.[21]

In North America, Indigenous youth are at particular risk for suicide. Suicide and self-inflicted injuries are the leading causes of death of First Nations and Inuit youth in Canada.[22] The most recent national data in Canada indicate that First Nations and Inuit youth ages fifteen to twenty-four are almost five to six times more likely to die by suicide than non-Indigenous youth. While there are no separate data for self-identified Métis youth, we know that suicide rates are approximately twice as high for self-identified Métis adults than for non-Indigenous people.[23] Suicide rates for Inuit youth are among the highest in the world, at eleven times the national average.[24] In the United States, the suicide rate among American Indian or Alaska Native (AIAN) youth is similarly elevated.[25, 26]

However, these suicide rates aren't inevitable. Rates vary between Indigenous communities and in those with lower rates, studies have shown that there are measures that may help reduce the number of completed suicides, such as self-government, land control, control over education, and higher rates of use of Indigenous languages, among others.[27, 28] Research indicating that suicide was rare in First Nations and Inuit communities prior to colonization also speaks to the latter's malevolent effects.

Forced assimilation, residential schools, mandatory community reloca-
tions, and the so-called Sixties Scoop, which saw Indigenous children
given to non-Indigenous parents for fostering and adoption, all led to
erosion of culture, traditional cultural values, and family integrity.[29, 30]

Trauma—a direct, witnessed, or learned-about experience of actual or threatened death, serious injury, or sexual violence—is another
major environmental risk factor for developing a mood disorder, and is
experienced by some of the vulnerable groups we have just mentioned.
Children may also experience trauma in the form of painful medical procedures (for very young children), animal bites, serious car accidents,
residential fires, acts of individual or mass violence, natural disasters, or
physical, emotional, and sexual abuse.[31] Child refugees, asylum seekers,
children in public care, homeless youth, children with disabilities, children who are bullied, youth living in communities characterized by high
levels of violence,[32] and incarcerated youth are all at higher risk for both
exposure to trauma and for developing depression.

Symptoms of post-traumatic stress disorder include nightmares; experiences of reliving the traumatic event; nervousness; brief periods of
losing touch with reality; detachment from loved ones and previously
pleasurable experiences; uncertainty about the future and thoughts of
dying young; irritability; aggressiveness; withdrawal; and headaches and
stomachaches. In younger children, trauma may cause regression to an
earlier developmental stage and behaviors such as thumb sucking, bed
wetting, and refusing to eat unless fed by a caregiver, like an infant. If
trauma is left untreated, it can lead to depression, substance misuse, broken relationships, and, tragically, sometimes suicide.[33, 34] In fact, three-
quarters of chronically depressed adults have histories of childhood
trauma,[35] and individuals with a mood disorder *and* a childhood history
of sexual or physical abuse have a significantly increased risk of death by
suicide.[36, 37]

It feels urgent to us—with youth suicide rates climbing—to point out the potential tragic impact of another environmental risk factor commonly experienced by young people: media coverage of suicide. In the past few years, explicit reporting of celebrity deaths by suicide has focused too often on the methods used and the reasons why the celebrity may have died in this manner—despite recommendations from mental health experts to avoid these areas of focus—instead of highlighting people who have successfully sought treatment and support in the face of suicidal thoughts. And it's not just the media. It's the entertainment industry as well. *13 Reasons Why*, a popular web-TV series that was criticized for seemingly glorifying the impact of a young girl's suicide on those who mistreated her, was associated with a spike in deaths by suicide among the show's target audience age group in the months following its release.[38, 39]

As parents, we want to protect our children from being exposed to these environmental factors, but the truth is, we can't shield them from everything. Daunting as this realization may be, it is good to know that understanding and being aware of our children's potential mental health risks are our best tools in mitigating their impact. After we look at the biological and psychological risk factors, we'll delve more deeply into what you can do to help prevent your child from developing a mood disorder, or to minimize its impact.

Biological Factors

As with other psychiatric disorders, genetics play a significant role in whether a child will develop a mood disorder.[40] A child whose parent has a depressive or substance use disorder is up to 24 percent more likely to develop depression.[41] Having an immediate relative with bipolar disorder makes a child seven times more likely than average to develop the disorder.[42]

There are also some medical disorders, particularly chronic medical illnesses—physical disabilities, neurodevelopmental disorders, traumatic brain injury, diseases involving the endocrine (hormonal) system, autoimmune disorders—that are all associated with an increased risk for children of developing depression.

Some medications increase a child's risk of developing a mood disorder, including antiseizure medications, stimulant medications used for ADHD, benzodiazepines, ibuprofen, the antibiotic ciprofloxacin, and some antidepressants themselves.[43] While this is not an exhaustive list, we have mentioned a few here so that you are aware of the potential side effects, especially if your child is already vulnerable because of family history.

Psychological Factors

Children who have emotionally reactive temperaments (quick to cry and to seek comfort, easily affected by day-to-day events), are highly self-critical and ruminative, or frequently get in trouble for disobedient behavior are at a higher risk for developing a mood disorder.[44] Children with learning disorders also appear to be at heightened risk, although this might be because of the social and academic pressures they face rather than vulnerability to the mood disorder itself.[45] Additionally, children with diagnoses of oppositional defiant disorder—a pervasive, long-standing pattern of anger, irritability, argumentativeness, defiance, and vindictiveness that causes distress and negative impacts for the child in his or her social and educational lives—are at increased risk for both anxiety and depression.[46]

There has been some debate within the mental health profession as to whether children with ADHD and other so-called disruptive behaviors may sometimes be misdiagnosed and, in fact, have early-onset bipolar disorder or pediatric bipolar disorder. While ADHD can increase the risk of a child's developing bipolar disorder later, we can't diagnose pediatric bipolar disorder without clear evidence of a pattern of episodic mood swings (not simply limited to irritability) with accompanying changes in sleep, behavior, energy, and thoughts.[47, 48] If your child has ADHD, and you are concerned you may be seeing such a pattern, we recommend you talk to your child's doctor.

What can parents do to prevent mood disorders and suicidal thoughts and behaviors?

While there are no guarantees, there are things you can do to lower the risk of your child developing a mood disorder and suicidal thoughts.

- Ensure children develop good sleep habits.
- Keep an eye out for any signs of bullying and intervene collaboratively with your child and his school. There are more and less effective ways to intervene, so seek education and help from experts, such as school board social workers and researchers in the field, if needed and share what you learn with your child's school.[49]
- Teach them—and yourselves!—how to reduce and manage stress.[50]
- Help children develop and foster personal strengths by introducing them to sports, hobbies, the arts, and so on.
- Help children develop social supports and coping strategies, including
  - a good sense of humor;
  - positive friendship networks; and
  - a close relationship with one or more family members.
- Make sure the lines of communication are open.
- Approach conflicts with your child in constructive ways; avoid criticizing and shouting, which tend to leave conflicts unresolved.
- Be aware of potential risk factors such as trauma and family history, and make sure your child receives treatment for related symptoms.

- If your child identifies as LGBTQ2S, support his or her or their identity! Research has demonstrated clearly that young people who have parental support for their sexual minority orientation or gender identity have significantly lower rates of mental health disorders and suicide.[51]

- Identify and treat any other psychiatric disorders your child may be struggling with, such as eating disorders and substance use disorders.

- Support policies and interventions that help youth mental health, particularly in high-risk areas such as Indigenous and LGBTQ2S communities. Given what we know about the contagion effects of high suicide rates in this age group, we need to protect our children regardless of background.[52]

- Keep any weapons or medications (including over-the-counter) out of reach of children, to prevent impulsive suicide attempts.

The most important thing you can do is make sure your relationship with your child is positive and supportive, even in times of conflict. If your child does develop mood symptoms or persistent irritability, open communication remains key. Many children tell us that they don't share suicidal thoughts with their mothers and fathers because they're worried that their parents will be devastated, blame themselves, or put them on lockdown. As parents, we understand the instinct to feel and do all of these things, especially when you're caught off guard and feel afraid for your child, but we encourage you to find the sweet spot between overreacting and underreacting. Tell your child that you love him, then listen. Don't move to "fix" the problem too quickly, as this prevents your child from telling you how he got to this desperate place, and he may perceive your response as uncaring or uninterested. We know that having these conversations is scary, and if you want advice on how to broach the topic of suicide with your son or daughter, we've included some resources at the end of the book.

When it comes to exposure to traumatic events and experiences, we remind you that no parent can prevent unforeseen tragedies. All we can do is teach our children that life can be unpredictable and sometimes painful, and remind them that it is our relationships, our coping strategies, time, and support networks that help us survive these tough experiences. If your child has experienced trauma, talk to her doctor about getting her the supports she needs as soon as possible. Here are a few other ways to reduce the likelihood and impact of childhood trauma:

- Have clear safety-related household rules.
- Monitor your child's activities but don't be controlling.
- Build a supportive family environment and social connections, including adults outside the family who can act as mentors.
- Ensure that your child has access to health care and community supports where possible, such as day care and school.[53, 54]
- Educate your child about her right to say no to others touching her body.
- Emphasize to your child the importance of speaking up to trusted adults if other children or adults hurt, sexually harass, or abuse him or her.

Remember, as parents, you can do everything right, and still your child may face these difficulties. Our hope is that these suggestions will help you and your child maintain a supportive relationship throughout hard times and prevent even worse outcomes.

Reaching a Diagnosis

Over the next few days, as Sara and Dror wait for Chana to wake up, they meet with various staff on the psychiatry team, including Dr. Isabel Rodrigues, the psychiatrist responsible for Chana's care while she is in hospital, and Ron Lee, the social worker, who tells them what to expect in the coming days. After suggesting reading materials and support groups for them to explore, Ron, whose friendliness and invitation to use his first name immediately endear him to Sara, encourages them to maintain as much of Chana's privacy as they can and to refrain from sharing details with her friends, family, and school until she is able to express her preferences about who can be informed. Both Sara and Dror find Ron's practicality reassuring.

Finally, on the third day, when Sara is trying to work from home, she gets the call telling her that Chana has woken up. She rushes to the hospital to find her daughter sitting up in bed with a tube taped to her left nostril and intravenous lines attached to two poles. Chana is pale and looks at least five years younger than she did when she left for the party last Saturday that preceded her suicide attempt, but she's conscious. And she's alive.

Sara leans in to kiss Chana. "My poor girl. My poor, lovely girl. I am so sorry you felt this terrible, and I didn't know and didn't help." Tears roll down both their faces.

"Mom, I'm sorry." Chana's voice is raspy as a result of having been intubated. "I couldn't talk to you about how I was feeling. I didn't want you to worry."

Sara stops herself from asking how Chana thought keeping her secret and hurting herself wouldn't make Sara worry. She simply squeezes Chana's hand. "I love you, Chana." Her daughter is like a precious piece of glass, and she's afraid she could break her with a rough touch.

Just then Dr. Rodrigues enters the room.

"I'm glad to see you are doing better, Chana," she says kindly. "The nurse tells me you are feeling much more alert and would like to talk to me on your own." She turns to Sara. "I can come back later, though, if you'd like a little more time together."

Sara feels a stab of sadness that Chana prefers to talk to someone other than her about what drove her to attempt suicide, but she's also a bit relieved. She's not sure she's ready to hear what her daughter has to say. Sara gives Chana a tentative hug. "I'll be right outside in the family lounge."

"Thanks, Mom," Chana croaks.

Forty-five minutes later, a volunteer tells Sara that Chana and Dr. Rodrigues would like to see her. Sara can tell that Chana has been crying—there are crumpled tissues on the pale-blue bedcover—but she seems more relaxed.

"Chana's been incredibly brave and honest," Dr. Rodrigues says. "Over the past months, she's experienced symptoms of depression, but we've agreed that it is important for her to tell you what happened. I'm here to help her if she has difficulty."

Sara moves her chair to the bed and takes Chana's cool hand in hers. "Love, there isn't anything you can't tell me."

Chana starts to talk, her gaze fixed on the psychiatrist and away from Sara. Haltingly, she tells her mother that she was sexually assaulted by a couple of boys from her school at a party last semester. She was unconscious from drinking at the time and only found out later that they had taken naked pictures of themselves raping her and circulated them on social media.

Sara feels nauseated and light-headed. She grips the arms of her chair tightly and reminds herself to breathe. She looks to Dr. Rodrigues. What can she possibly say that will help her daughter right now? That will help Sara?

Dr. Rodrigues's voice is calm. "Chana, I can only imagine how difficult it is to talk about this. The sexual assault took away your sense of control and privacy. It's important we give you back a sense of your boundaries. Disclosing what was done to you was a first step towards recovery. Now you can get the support you need to start to heal."

"My love. I am so desperately sorry this happened to you. Why couldn't you tell me?" Sara asks, her voice unsteady.

"Mom, I've been so ashamed. I thought you would be so disappointed in me. I'm sorry, Mom. I'm a terrible daughter." By now, Chana is crying, and all Sara can do is hold her and stroke her hair, and tell her that she loves her, that she is her best girl and a wonderful daughter, and that everything—everything—will be okay.

For the first time in many months, Sara hugs her daughter, and Chana hugs her back.

When Chana's sobs die down, Sara tentatively asks a question she has been dreading:

"Why did you take those pills, Chana?"

Chana looks to Dr. Rodrigues, who speaks again. "Chana tells me that she has been trying to self-medicate her depression and PTSD with alcohol. She was drinking at the party last Saturday when she saw one of the boys who assaulted her. She was overwhelmed by the memories of what had happened, and when she came home, she took all the pills she could find in the house."

Sara rubs her daughter's hand. "Oh, Chana. I'm so, so sorry."

"I'll let you two spend some time alone together now. Chana's sharing what happened to her is both courageous and an essential step in her recovery. In our experience, when adolescents who harm themselves keep secrets from their parents out of shame or fear of rejection, they are more likely to increase their self-harm and other high-risk behaviors until they have shared their burdens." Dr. Rodrigues adds gently, "We still have to confirm Chana's diagnosis and decide on next steps and treatment, but we have time. Chana's agreed to stay in the psychiatry unit for a few days after she's finished her treatment in the ICU." The psychiatrist turns to Chana.

"You were very brave today. Don't forget how strong you are."

Sara looks at her daughter and hopes that she is strong enough to help Chana through whatever comes next. She also makes a mental note to ask Dr. Rodrigues about whether charging the boys who did this would help Chana.

What are the treatments for mood disorders?

The above vignette is an example of what parents might expect if faced with a terrifying reality such as Sara's and Chana's. We did not show the step-by-step process of confirming Chana's diagnosis of depression, but it would be similar to what we've discussed in previous chapters. Her doctors would run various tests to rule out any medical causes, and Chana and her mother would fill out questionnaires to confirm her diagnosis. While it is tempting to see Chana's trauma as the source of her depression, there are likely other factors, such as her father's death and her mother's depression. The trauma undoubtedly accelerated her symptoms and led her to try to end her life. However, it is important to emphasize that not every child with a mood disorder who attempts suicide has a history of trauma or an obvious reason for his or her attempt; in many cases, the distorted thinking that accompanies depression, and sometimes mania, is the only identifiable cause. Regardless of the causes, treatment will involve a variety of approaches to tackle each issue the child is struggling with.

When anyone attempts suicide, the first step is to devise a safety plan, which includes removing anything in the house that the child can use to end her life and improving her communication with the support people in her life. Given that no environment can be entirely safety proofed, it's essential that parents talk to their children about whom they can turn to when they experience sadness and dark thoughts. For children who find it difficult to discuss their suicidal thoughts and feelings directly, we recommend they create a verbal code of colors or numbers to alert their support people when they are in trouble. When a parent checks in about how the child feels, the child answers with a code or number with preassigned meaning and actions for parents (such as providing comfort or distraction or, if necessary, helping their child to seek crisis support). The safety plan also includes identifying helpful distractions and people the child feels comfortable spending time with when she feels sad or suicidal, in order to reduce social isolation and time spent alone ruminating.

The next step is to treat any underlying mood disorder or PTSD symptoms through education, psychotherapy, and, if necessary, medication.

Education

This aspect of treatment involves teaching children and their families about mood disorders, the impact of trauma if relevant, triggers for mood episodes, and strategies to prevent the frequency and severity of symptoms. We encourage children to develop healthy routines: to get enough sleep; eat right; exercise; cut back on drug use—if not stopping altogether—including cannabis and alcohol; and to focus on their own goals and hopes to inspire them to make the changes they need to get better.

Education can occur with individual families or in larger groups. Usually adolescents prefer to receive education on their own or with others their age rather than with their parents so that they can ask questions about subjects they are usually reluctant to talk about in front of their parents, such as substance use and sexuality.

Psychotherapies

There are many effective therapies available for children and teens struggling with mood disorders, and your child's doctor will be able to tell you which ones will work best for your child. Some target depression and others, bipolar disorder, but each has a slightly different focus, so your child's doctor may suggest that your family enroll in different treatments at different stages, depending on what your child needs at a given time. Most therapies last anywhere from five to twenty sessions, depending on the type and severity of the symptoms. We have summarized the different therapies for you in the table on the following pages.

Type of Therapy	Disorder	Recommended Age Group
Cognitive behavior therapy (CBT)	Depression, anxiety	Children and adolescents
Child- and family-focused cognitive behavior therapy (CFF-CBT)	Bipolar disorder	Younger children (8–12)
Trauma-focused cognitive behavior therapy	Post-traumatic stress disorder (PTSD) (May be used for other psychiatric disorders for which CBT is known to be effective but where trauma is also present.)	Children and adolescents
Interpersonal therapy (IPT)	Depression	Adolescents

Focus	Family's Role
Targets the relationship between thoughts, emotions, and behaviors. May be both a primary treatment or adjunctive (used in conjunction with medication and other therapies), depending on the severity of symptoms and their response to therapy alone.	Younger children generally see their therapist alone or in a group, while their parents learn the parenting-focused skills in their own sessions. Adolescents are usually seen alone, too, and they decide how much feedback their therapist will give parents.
Integrates traditional CBT with education, interpersonal therapy (IPT), and mindfulness strategies.[55] Adjunctive rather than primary treatment.	Family-based approach. Often multi-family format.
Tailored to take into consideration the role that trauma played in causing depressive symptoms.[56]	Therapy sessions can be one-on-one between the child and the therapist; or with child, parents, and therapists; or in a group setting with other children suffering from similar trauma.
Focuses through group therapy on how teens engage with others and the behaviors that cause isolation and frustration, and that lead to depressive symptoms. Therapists help the teen recognize these behaviors and develop better communication and relationship skills.[57] May be both a primary treatment or used in conjunction with medication and other therapies, depending on the severity of symptoms and their response to therapy alone.	The family's role is primarily supportive, and if education/support for the family is required, it will occur outside the adolescent's therapy.

Type of Therapy	Disorder	Recommended Age Group
Dialectical behavior therapy (DBT)	Repetitive self-harm or suicidal thoughts; bipolar disorder	Children and adolescents
Individual psychoeducation and multifamily psychoeducation groups[59, 60, 61]	Bipolar disorder	Young children and their parents
Family-focused therapy (FFT)	Bipolar disorder	Adolescents

Focus	Family's Role
Combines elements of CBT with traditional Eastern meditative practices to teach patients how to manage their emotions and replace self-destructive coping strategies with more adaptive ones. Teens learn to sit with intense and difficult emotions instead of pushing them away, to change damaging and unhelpful emotions, to focus on the present instead of painful episodes in the past, to communicate their relationship needs clearly, and to set boundaries with others while maintaining relationships. Adjunctive rather than primary treatment when used in bipolar disorder.[58]	Some DBT programs for children and adolescents have parent groups in which parents are encouraged to learn how to communicate with their teens, manage their own emotions in the face of their child's high-risk behaviors, and support their child when he or she struggles with self-harm and suicidal thoughts and impulses.
Provides parents with education about pediatric bipolar disorder and helps them learn how to manage their child's symptoms, while teaching children coping strategies.[62] Adjunctive rather than primary treatment.	Therapy sessions can involve individual families or groups of families. Therapy sessions are highly structured, with homework and group exercises and tasks.
Provides education to parents and teens, and uses elements of family therapy. FFT has been shown to hasten recovery from episodes of illness, lessen recurrences, and decrease symptom severity.[63] It's particularly effective when used with medication after an episode of acute illness. Adjunctive rather than primary treatment.	The entire family—patient, parents, and siblings—participates in FFT. Participants learn about bipolar disorder, communication skills, and problem solving.

Medications

For children with depression, the primary medications used in treatment are the SSRIs we discussed in our chapter on anxiety disorders. Of all the SSRIs, fluoxetine (Prozac) has the most research supporting its effectiveness in treating depression in children and adolescents, although there is more evidence to support its treatment for anxiety than depression in these age groups. Given this fact, any discussion of fluoxetine's use for child and adolescent depression requires an analysis of risk and benefit for each child. Some adolescents do not respond to fluoxetine or they experience intolerable side effects, in which event doctors may prescribe an alternative SSRI such as escitalopram (Lexapro) or sertraline (Zoloft). Both have studies to support their relative safety and effectiveness, and are FDA-approved in the United States, although not by Health Canada. Physicians may use "off-label" medications where there is sufficient evidence with regard to both safety and effectiveness to support a medication being used in children and adolescents, despite formal approval not having been sought by a pharmaceutical company or still being in process. Where this is the case, physicians should make families aware.

For children with depression, one of the important aspects of medication parents need to be aware of is that all antidepressant medications carry a risk of inducing a manic episode, a risk that is significantly higher in those with a family history of bipolar disorder. (In those cases, we try to avoid the use of medication if possible and focus instead on therapy.) If therapy alone proves insufficient, pharmacological treatment for depression in children at increased risk for bipolar disorder may involve the use of other families of medications such as atypical antipsychotics and mood stabilizers.

For children who have definitively been diagnosed with bipolar disorder, atypical antipsychotics, such as risperidone (Risperdal) and quetiapine (Seroquel), and mood stabilizers, such as lithium (Lithobid, Lithium Carbolith) and valproic acid (Depakene, Epival), are the two classes of medications used in treatment. They have good evidence supporting their effectiveness, but they do require careful monitoring, as they have significant potential medical side effects.

Long-term Care

While mood disorders are episodic in nature and respond well to treatment, the risk of recurrence is high. According to one of the largest and most rigorous treatment studies of adolescent depression, rates of recovery were approximately 88 percent within two years and 96 percent within five, but just under half of those teens who recovered experienced a further episode within five years. Young women[64] and patients with coexisting anxiety disorders were the most vulnerable to these recurrences. Bipolar disorder has a much higher risk of recurrent episodes over a lifetime—more than 90 percent, according to a large study of adults with the disorder.[65] Accordingly, parents need to be proactive and continue to work with their children on coping strategies in between acute episodes to protect against relapse.

After Treatment

During Chana's weeklong hospital stay, she completed her safety plan and identified Sara, Dror, and her uncle Ben as key support people, and her school guidance counsellor and grandparents as secondary supports. Her safety plan includes strategies and support if she encounters either of the boys who assaulted her. Although Chana agreed to inform her school that she had been hospitalized, in order for her to receive accommodation for the work she has missed, she did not want to share any more details, except with her guidance counsellor. Dr. Rodrigues talked with her about taking the antidepressant fluoxetine to treat her depressive and post-traumatic stress symptoms. So far, Chana has resisted. Sara has tried to remain supportive of this decision, but part of her thinks anything that will prevent a future suicide attempt is worth trying. The good news is that Chana has agreed to undergo cognitive behavior therapy following her discharge.

The best meetings during Chana's hospital stay involved Sara, Chana, and Dror. Together they revisited the loss of Max. Sara learned that both her children felt a need to protect her in the wake of their father's death, but they would like her to meet a new partner so they don't feel guilty leaving her alone when they go off to college.

While Chana didn't want to discuss the assault in detail, she did talk about how it made her feel. Telling Sara and Dror, painful as it was, helped. Chana hasn't decided if she wants to press charges. It's up to her whether or not to pursue this option because, from a legal perspective, at her age she is no longer considered a child in need of protection. Sara has to work hard not to pressure her; she would love to see the boys who did this to her daughter stand trial, but she's conscious of Chana's vulnerability in revisiting the trauma. They have had open conversations about the dangers of alcohol and drugs. Both Sara and Dror told Chana what she means to them and how unbearable her loss would be for them.

On the day of Chana's discharge from the hospital, they have their final team meeting in the usual drab, sparsely furnished unit family room. Chana, dressed in her favorite torn jeans and a bright orange sweater that Sara hasn't seen her wear for months, asks when she can go back to school.

"I know it's going to be brutal," she acknowledges, "but I think I'm ready for it. I probably won't go back there for grade twelve, but I think I can get through the rest of this year, especially with the accommodations they've agreed to put in place for me to catch up. And I know who my true friends are now." She pauses as a shadow crosses her face. "And if it doesn't work out, if I can't handle it, I just need to speak up."

Dror puts his arm around her. "That's right, you do. And who says you need to get through high school in four years? Lots of people take victory laps these days. If it turns out to be too much, we'll figure it out."

Chana hugs him back, and Sara's heart warms at the sight. At the end of the session, she stays behind when her two children go to get Chana's suitcase from the nursing station. She turns to Dr. Rodrigues.

"How will I keep her safe? How will I know if she is slipping?"

"There are no guarantees in life," the doctor replies, "but you've educated yourself on the warning signs, and you've proven to her that you're strong enough to support her through trauma. No parent can do more; the rest is up to Chana. I know that's terrifying, but this crisis has also changed her and taught her many things about herself and the strength of her family."

Sara draws a deep breath and takes Dr. Rodrigues's hand.

"Thank you. For not pretending everything will be easy and for helping all of us to reconnect with one another."

As Sara leaves the hospital with her daughter and son, she knows in her gut that they are more tightly connected now than they were before.

Bipolar Disorders

Disorder	Description
Bipolar I disorder	Defined by manic episodes that last at least seven days, or by manic symptoms that are so severe that the person needs immediate hospital care. Usually depressive episodes occur as well, typically lasting at least two weeks. Episodes of depression with mixed features (having depression and manic symptoms at the same time) are also possible.
Bipolar II disorder	Defined by a pattern of depressive episodes and hypomanic episodes, but not the full-blown manic episodes described above.
Cyclothymic disorder (cyclothymia)	Defined by numerous periods of some hypomanic symptoms as well as numerous periods lasting at least one year of some depressive symptoms in children and adolescents (two years in adults), but not enough for a diagnosis of actual hypomanic or depressive episodes.

Psychosis

A Child in Distress

Liz digs through her cluttered purse, looking for her ringing cell phone. The ring tone is a rap song her seventeen-year-old son, Blake, downloaded last summer. She really should get rid of it, she thinks now, finally locating the blaring device, but she loves how Blake grins every time he hears it.

"Hello?" she says.

"Is this Ms. Fadden?" The woman on the other end sounds official.

"Yes, speaking."

"This is Police Sergeant Shah, calling from Niagara. Are you the mother of Blake Fadden?"

Liz's heart is in her mouth. "Yes. Is he okay?"

"We have Blake here with us. He seems physically fine, apart from being hungry, but he's not making a lot of sense."

"I don't understand. Blake is supposed to be at school."

"Ms. Fadden, he got on the bus to Niagara Falls this morning and attempted to cross into the United States, but he wouldn't talk to the border guards about the purpose of his trip. He kept repeating it had to be confidential."

Liz can feel hot tears dripping down her cheeks, but she tries to keep her voice steady. "I need to call my husband at work. We'll come right away."

"We are going to take Blake to the nearest hospital to be assessed by a psychiatrist. Please join us there."

"Of course. We'll leave now. Let me just take down the location."

The entire car ride to Niagara, Liz and her husband, Richard, are lost in their own thoughts. Over the past couple of weeks, Blake has talked about being under surveillance by the US government, but they chalked it up to a combination of his fascination with Internet stories about hackers, and stress from being in his final year of high school and applying to universities. They thought he might be smoking pot, but he never appeared to be high or smelled like cannabis. Now as they drive, they wonder if they should have been more worried sooner. Normally gregarious, Blake had withdrawn from his siblings and friends over the past six months and spent most of his time hanging out in the basement playing video games, scrolling through news feeds, or writing in an ever-growing pile of lined notebooks that he possessively told them were top secret. Their seventeen-year-old was having trouble sleeping, too. Liz and Richard tried to get him to see their family doctor, but every time they brought it up, he said he was fine and too busy to go. Richard wanted to press the issue, but Liz didn't want Blake to think they were ganging up on him.

Now she broods over what stopped her from following up. Was there some part of her that was afraid there might be a more serious problem? If she had made Blake go to the doctor, would they be where they are right now?

At the emergency department, a nurse ushers them to their son's room and lets them know that Dr. Andrew Law, the on-call psychiatrist, will be along shortly. In the meantime, a crisis worker is with Blake. Liz can't help but notice that a security guard also sits outside the door. The room itself is windowless, and there is no medical equipment. A woman sitting with Blake rises from her seat and introduces herself as Sharon, the crisis worker. Liz nods at her, but her breath catches when she sees Blake curled up on one of the orange vinyl love seats, scribbling furiously on a pad of paper. His plaid shirt is open at the collar, revealing protruding clavicles, and his dirty jeans have multiple holes. How had she not realized how thin he'd become? Liz goes to him, but he flinches when she hugs him, consumed with his writing.

"Hey, Blakie." Richard's voice, usually forceful, is gentle as he squeezes his son's shoulder. "You gave your mother and me quite a surprise. You haven't been to Niagara Falls since we came in ninth grade with the hockey team. I knew you liked the Clifton Hill arcades, but not this much . . ."

Blake pauses and looks up uncertainly. "Sorry, Dad. I only decided to make this trip this morning."

"We're just glad you're safe."

There is a quiet knock on the doorframe, and Liz and Richard turn to see a tall man—who to their eyes doesn't look much older than Blake—enter the room.

"This is Dr. Law," Sharon says. "He'll be able to answer your questions."

Dr. Law closes the door and comes over to shake Liz's and Richard's hands. He nods at Blake and explains that he and Blake have spoken at length and he has permission to discuss their conversation with Liz and Richard. Blake once again focuses on his writing.

"Is our son okay?" Richard asks.

"Physically, yes. I have told Blake that it's his mental state that we're concerned about. Blake has told us he is worried about a conspiracy and that US intelligence operatives are after him. He was scared at first that we might be part of the plot, but we seem to have reassured him that this is a safe place and we're here to help him figure things out."

Liz exchanges a look with Richard. They had no idea their son was suffering from such bizarre beliefs. "Do you have any idea of what's causing this?" she asks.

"I have explained to Blake that I believe that he has lost touch with reality and is experiencing paranoia and hallucinations. The medical term for what he is experiencing is a psychotic episode."

At the word *psychotic*, Liz feels herself sway and leans on Richard for support. No, this can't be happening, she thinks.

"I understand this is a shock," Dr. Law continues. "Right now the important thing to focus on is the fact that Blake is safe and willing to accept our help to figure this out. Now that we know something is wrong, we can get him the help he needs. And we will. We're running a few tests now, but once those are done, we'll have Blake transferred to a hospital nearer to your home."

"Thank you, Doctor," Richard says, squeezing Liz's hand, but his wife is in a daze. She studies her son. Where is the outgoing boy who made a raucous song her ringtone? Will they ever get him back? Will he be able to go back to school, attend college, get married? Will he struggle for the rest of his life? Her mind wanders to the people she sees on her way to work downtown every morning, bedraggled, sometimes shouting, talking to themselves, always alone. These are the people she thought about when the psychiatrist said the word *psychotic*. But this is Blake, her baby. She won't let that happen to him.

What is psychosis?

The above vignette is an example of how a child suffering from psychosis might behave and what a psychotic episode might look like to his or her parents. Liz's reaction to hearing the words *psychotic episode* is completely normal. It's a scary diagnosis. And like Liz, many of us associate psychosis with images of isolated, unstable people either on the street or in mental institutions. In fact, long-term psychotic disorders are relatively rare compared with a discrete experience of psychotic symptoms. While approximately three in one hundred people will have a psychotic episode during their lifetime,[1] of those, far fewer will develop a long-term psychotic disorder.[2] In other words, a single psychotic episode doesn't mean a lifetime diagnosis. Research studies indicate that up to 17 percent of children ages nine through twelve and 7.5 percent of adolescents report experiencing some psychotic symptoms, but only a small number of those children will go on to develop a chronic psychotic disorder.[3]

But if you and your child are facing the possibility that he or she has psychotic symptoms, statistics and likelihoods don't always feel helpful. When it comes to your own child, you need specific questions answered. In that instance, we recommend you speak with your child's doctor as soon as possible. For more general questions about psychosis and its treatment, we hope to be able to answer those in this chapter. Below we'll walk you through exactly what psychosis is and what you can expect if your child is diagnosed with psychotic symptoms. We'll also discuss schizophrenia, a longer-term psychotic disorder, which could be one of the possible causes for their symptoms. And in the back of the book, you'll find a list of helpful resources.

First, psychosis itself is not a disorder; it is a set of symptoms caused by a neuropsychiatric syndrome characterized by a malfunction in the development of interconnected neural networks within and between the frontal and temporal regions of the brain. All that means is that these parts of the brain aren't communicating with each other effectively. This can be temporary or permanent. Since the frontal and temporal lobes are responsible for interpreting what we experience in the world around us,[4] when there's a problem, we lose our ability to distinguish between what is real and what is not. In other words, innocent sensory triggers are misinterpreted as dangerous. For Blake, that meant he initially thought that the customs officials at the border were part of a sinister surveillance squad.

Specific symptoms of psychosis can include:

- hallucinations, where the person sees, hears, feels, tastes, or smells things that are not present;
- delusions (fixed irrational beliefs) about what is happening to and around the person, which may cause him paranoia or to think he has special powers;
- disorganized and incoherent thinking, speech, behavior, and emotional reactions;
- impaired sleep, concentration, and memory;
- mood changes and suicidal feelings; and
- social withdrawal, lack of motivation, and difficulty initiating ideas and tasks, all of which mental health professionals refer to as negative symptoms, in contrast to the previous effects, which are called positive symptoms.

If your adolescent is exhibiting one or more of these symptoms, or if you notice other drastic changes in her behavior and routine, she may be suffering from a psychotic disorder, and we urge you to have her seen by a primary care physician and a psychiatrist as soon as possible. Left untreated, psychosis can become extraordinarily debilitating, leading to deteriorating physical health, academic and vocational failure, broken relationships with friends and family, violence at the hands of others, substance use disorders, and, most concerning of all, suicide.

That said, often, especially in younger children, apparent psychotic symptoms are often caused by something more benign than a chronic psychotic disorder. Up to 66 percent of young children and approximately 30 percent to 40 percent of adolescents report occasional "psychotic-like experiences" (PLEs).[5, 6] A PLE occurs when someone believes that an object, action, or circumstance not logically related to a course of events can influence its outcome.[7] For example, truly believing that black cats bring bad luck and taking extraordinary measures to avoid them is a PLE. But sometimes, what may seem like a PLE could merely be masking garden-variety disobedience. A child of five or six who blames his bad behavior on hearing voices but shows no drastic changes in behavior, mood, or communication likely isn't suffering from a psychotic disorder. In fact, in our opinion, it's often a sign he's able to think his way out of a tough situation! Below we've included a few other scenarios that, if your child is otherwise well, are completely normal:

- Children age ten and under who have imaginary friends. In time, they will say goodbye.
- Children who believe in ghosts and an afterlife, and who report seeing presences in their home, especially when others in the family discuss supernatural phenomena.
- Children who see or hear a loved one after death. This is a common experience during the early stages of bereavement.
- Children who imagine a shape or figure, or hear a voice in the twilight between waking and sleeping. These are normal experiences known as hypnopompic and hypnagogic hallucinations.
- Children who misinterpret a curtain or a coat stand as a person, or a sound as a voice or threat. These are common perceptual illusions.

Other situations give cause for greater concern, such as when other mental health issues resemble or contribute to psychotic symptoms. For example, children suffering from PTSD may experience flashbacks that mimic psychotic symptoms.[8,9] And as we mentioned in our previous chapter, those suffering from a mood disorder may have delusions that border on psychosis. For instance, individuals with mania may believe that they are famous, fabulously rich, or have special talents or magical powers, while someone with depression may believe he has lost all his money, or suffers from a terrible illness, or has committed a crime.[10] Some children with obsessive-compulsive disorder experience their intrusive thoughts as voices. Some prescription medications and recreationally used substances can also cause psychosis. In each of these scenarios, your child's doctor will work with you and your child to uncover what's causing his psychotic symptoms and get him the help he needs.

What are the different types of psychotic disorders and their warning signs?

All psychotic disorders share the same warning signs—in other words, the various symptoms of psychosis, positive or negative—described above. Depending on the specific cause of your child's psychotic symptoms, she may experience symptoms for a few hours, a couple of days, or several weeks, or she may experience symptoms for much longer, up to and beyond six months.

The causes of psychosis can be categorized into a few broad areas: (1) medical conditions such as an infection, a tumor, or an autoimmune disorder that attacks the brain; (2) prescription, nonprescription, and recreational drugs; and (3) psychiatric disorders. With both medical conditions and drugs, symptoms develop quite quickly, but with psychiatric disorders, symptoms usually, although not always, emerge over time.

As we mentioned earlier, up to 30 percent of people who experience a psychotic episode never have another.[11] For individuals whose initial symptoms last less than six months and who receive treatment and show no further symptoms, the likelihood that they will have an improved overall level of functioning long term and not experience recurrences is significantly greater than for individuals with a chronic psychotic disorder such as schizophrenia.[12] In our experience, schizophrenia is one of the most frightening diagnoses for teens and their parents to contemplate, and so we briefly discuss it below to assuage some of those fears.

Schizophrenia

Schizophrenia is a chronic psychotic disorder, which means that the person has experienced psychotic symptoms for at least a month and impaired functioning as a result for at least six months. And while there may be periods of relief from active psychosis, the sufferer's level of functioning in between acute episodes usually never fully recovers to where it was prior to the onset of the illness. It is important for parents to know that schizophrenia is relatively rare. Despite difficulties collecting accurate data on how common schizophrenia is (because of differences in how different international studies define and diagnose it), we know that it is much rarer than the other, shorter-lived psychotic disorders described previously. Recent estimates suggest that less than three-quarters of 1 percent of people will be diagnosed with schizophrenia during their lifetimes (i.e., less than 75 out of 10,000 individuals), but the number drops significantly for children under the age of thirteen, to one in ten thousand.[13, 14, 15] The likelihood increases slightly for children between the ages of thirteen and eighteen, and then more dramatically for young men in their late teens and early twenties, and for women about a decade later.

We understand that the idea of your child suffering from a chronic psychotic illness can be overwhelming, but we know from patients and families that schizophrenia is not a death sentence. There are a number of effective treatments and psychosocial interventions to manage the symptoms and to minimize the negative aspects of the disease, particularly the risks of social isolation and vocational setbacks, so that your child can live a fulfilling life.

What are the risk factors for developing a psychotic disorder?

Environmental and Psychological Factors

The known environmental risks for developing psychosis overlap with psychological factors: childhood histories of immigration (and particularly refugee status),[16] trauma, exposure to adversity, and living in an urban center[17] (which doubles a child's risk compared with living in a rural area[18]). These factors are obviously multifaceted in nature, and it is extremely challenging for researchers to tease out which factors predispose an individual to psychosis. In the mental health profession, we've theorized that when young children experience these environmental factors, the associated stress affects their developing brains in ways that we don't yet have the science to understand fully.

Carbon monoxide poisoning and heavy metal contamination from substances such as lead may seem like ancient risks, but lead pipes remain an issue in older homes. Exposure can lead to neurodevelopmental disorders and, in extreme cases, hallucinations.[19, 20] While these are rare occurrences today in North America, the possibility should be considered once other causes for psychosis have been ruled out and when a child has lived for the past six months in a house or apartment built before 1960 (especially if the house is being renovated, water is supplied by lead pipes, or original paint is present, peeling, or chipped). It's also worth considering in instances where the child emigrated or was internationally adopted from a country where the population is exposed to more lead than in Canada and the United States.[21]

Biological Factors

Genetics are a significant risk factor for developing a psychotic disorder. Children with a parent or sibling with schizophrenia are 9 percent more likely to develop schizophrenia or another psychotic disorder than the general population,[22] with identical twins at a lifetime risk of more than 40 percent.[23] Additionally, children with autism are at greater risk for developing both bipolar disorder and schizophrenia in adulthood.[24]

In terms of other biological factors, as we mentioned above, certain medical illnesses such as genetic or inherited errors of metabolism, which affect how children's bodies break down nutritional compounds, can cause psychosis to develop in childhood, as can tumors, infections, and autoimmune disorders. Delirium—a brain condition that can occur at any age and has multiple causes—can resemble psychosis, producing confusion, lack of awareness of time and place, agitation or lethargy (sometimes alternating), and hallucinations.

Difficulties in a mother's pregnancy and during birth—particularly intrauterine malnutrition and growth retardation, loss of oxygen to the baby, and prenatal stress or infection—have been shown to increase a child's risk of developing schizophrenia prior to adulthood.[25] In any of these scenarios, the baby may suffer injuries that make him or her more susceptible to problems with brain development,[26] perhaps leading to specific vulnerabilities in the brain that have been associated with the presence of psychotic symptoms.

The abuse of alcohol and recreational drugs such as cocaine, amphetamine, methamphetamine, LSD, MDMA, cannabis, magic mushrooms, and ketamine can all increase the risk of psychosis. In children and teens, these substances, particularly cannabis when used daily and in high potency formulations, directly affect brain development.[27, 28]

What can parents do to prevent psychosis?

Unlike some other mental illnesses, we simply don't know enough yet about most of the causes of psychosis to know how best to prevent them. Having said that, we encourage you to talk to your children about the risks of misusing prescription medications and recreational substances, particularly cannabis, which are modifiable risk factors. And if you have a family history of psychosis, watch closely for signs and symptoms.

Remember, you know your child better than anyone, and if his behavior and attitude change markedly, don't be afraid to seek professional help. While there might not be much you can do to prevent the disease, some preliminary evidence suggests that early intervention for individuals exhibiting features of psychosis has a positive impact on their outcome. These initial steps include education about psychosis for the individual and family; improving health-related behaviors such as sleep, exercise, and nutrition; individual therapy such as CBT; family engagement; and planning crisis support such as when to use emergency medical services or to consider hospitalization in the event of an acute relapse and/or safety concerns for the individual or others.[29]

Reaching a Diagnosis

The next morning, Liz and Richard arrive at their local hospital. Blake is staying in the psychiatry ward, and Liz notices that each room along the hallway has a wall of thick Plexiglas. When they enter Blake's room, she sees that there's no furniture other than a low bed, a built-in cupboard, and a small desk, where a breakfast tray sits untouched.

Blake is pacing, but rushes towards them. "I can't stay here. It doesn't feel safe. I need to go home."

The look in his eye scares Liz. "I'm afraid the doctors need you to stay here for a few more days," she says quickly. "We need to get you help."

The nurse sitting nearby introduces herself as Rula Mohammed. "It's actually up to Blake whether he stays," she says gently. "He's a voluntary patient."

Liz is shocked. How can anyone think of letting him go in this state?

The nurse guides Liz over to the corner of the room. "I know it's hard, but the doctors have assessed that Blake isn't a threat to himself or others. We recommend that parents take the long view. It's important to give him autonomy and choice so that he doesn't see treatment as something to escape from but something he chooses. And it is a good sign he is okay with your coming to meetings with us. Not all our patients are comfortable with their parents being involved."

Liz nods, but she is unconvinced. They will know more soon. Blake met with Dr. Vera Krishnev, his inpatient psychiatrist, this morning, and they have a follow-up family meeting with her in a half hour.

"I want to go home," Blake says again.

"Hey, bud, let's talk about this," Richard says. "Let's not make a sudden decision. Why don't you finish your breakfast? I know I'm starving, and you must be hungrier than me. We can talk through the pros and cons while we eat."

"That's a great idea," Nurse Mohammed says. "How about you make a list, Blake?" She goes out of the room and returns with a pen and a pad of paper.

A look of confusion passes over Blake's face, as though he can't figure out what has been asked of him or how to form a response. After a few long moments, he nods his head. Richard sits next to Blake, and after taking the pen and paper from the nurse, hands them to his son. Liz stands farther back, instinctively not wanting to crowd them. She listens to Richard ask Blake if he can eat a few bites of his toast and suggest he write down his thoughts. After what seems like an eternity but is probably only about five or so minutes, Blake looks up at both the nurse and Liz.

"I think I will stay, at least for another day or two. The doctor said she'd like to start medication to help me feel better, and that's a good thing to do in hospital in case I have side effects." He turns back towards his breakfast tray, offers Richard a slice of toast, and starts to eat himself.

"I think that's a good decision," Richard says. "Thanks for the toast. It's not bad."

Liz feels a surge of gratitude towards her husband for his level, unruffled approach.

Once Blake finishes his breakfast, the nurse escorts the three of them to a small, equally sparse meeting room down the hall. Dr. Krishnev, a petite woman in her early forties, introduces herself to Liz and Richard, shaking their hands. The younger woman next to her does the same and tells them her name is Inez Ramos, the team social worker. She says she'll be working closely with them going forward through treatment.

"Hello again, Blake," Dr. Krishnev says, her voice quiet and interested. "How are you feeling now that you've had breakfast and a chance to speak with your parents?"

He takes a moment to respond, as though he's bringing his attention back from a far place. "Better. I talked to my dad, and I've decided to stay in hospital for a couple more days."

"Good, I'm glad you came to that decision." She smiles. "We have a lot to talk about today, and I'd like to start with what happens next. Is that okay with you?"

Blake nods, his gaze drifting to the window.

Dr. Krishnev explains that the hospital in Niagara has sent over questionnaires that Liz and Richard completed in the emergency department about Blake's recent behavior as well as the results of his physical exam and blood and urine tests. "The team here will follow up with a few more specific tests, but so far they haven't found any potential medical causes for Blake's psychotic episode."

Liz's face falls. She wishes the cause of her son's illness was an easily eradicable piece of his body that could be cut out, like an appendix. Then this nightmare would be over, and they could all go back to the way things were.

Dr. Krishnev continues. "Nothing has shown up on Blake's initial tests that indicates he has a neurological disorder or an infection or inflammatory process in the brain. He hasn't had any seizures, unusual body movements, visual disturbances, numbness, or visual or olfactory hallucinations—*olfactory* is a bit technical; it simply means when someone detects a smell that isn't present in their environment. The emergency department in Niagara took a computerized tomography, or CT, scan, which allowed us to view Blake's brain in cross-sections, using a computerized series of X-rays from all directions. Everything looked normal, which is good. There was nothing to suggest any structural abnormalities, bleeds, or tumors that might be contributing to his symptoms."[30] She pauses, allowing time for them to ask further questions. Blake shows no interest, continuing to stare out the window.

"Blake, is there anything needing your attention right now?"

He nods without breaking his gaze. "The voices," he says.

Liz feels her mouth go dry.

"Blake, can I share with your parents what you told me about the voices this morning?"

His eyes refocus, and he looks at the doctor. "Okay."

Dr. Krishnev turns to Richard and Liz. "For the past several months, Blake has been hearing voices, telling him that he is being poisoned by electronic laser beams orchestrated by the US Intelligence Services." She turns back to Blake. "What are they saying to you now?"

"They're reminding me I have a lot to do, and that being in the hospital is getting in the way of my research. If I can't figure out how I'm being monitored by the Pentagon, my whole family is in danger."

Liz searches for Richard's hand. He squeezes hers back.

"Blake, thank you for explaining," Dr. Krishnev says calmly. "As we discussed this morning, our team thinks there's a strong possibility that your *perception* that you are under surveillance is the result of a brain illness."

Liz notices that the doctor hasn't contradicted Blake directly but merely offered an alternative explanation for what he is experiencing.

Dr. Krishnev addresses Liz and Richard. "We want to run a few more medical tests, but as I have said, so far there doesn't appear to be any medical explanation for Blake's symptoms. Given that, I have told him that we're fairly certain that he is suffering from what is called schizophreniform disorder. But we are not making a diagnosis of schizophrenia at this point. Blake's been experiencing his symptoms for around four months now, and for a diagnosis of schizophrenia to be made, he would have to have had symptoms for at least six months. He also doesn't seem to have had any associated mood symptoms that would point to other possible psychiatric disorders, but we will need to explore these issues further with all of you. In the interim, while we try to sort everything out, we would like to talk about treatment—exercise, sleep, talk therapy, and medication. I have already started to speak with Blake about these."

"How long will all of this take?" their son asks.

"I imagine it will take a couple of days to complete all the medical tests. And as you and I discussed, if we decide to start a medication to help with the confusion in your thinking, we would like you to stay a few more days to make sure that you feel okay on it and that we have you on the right dose. How does that sound?"

"So, about a week?"

"Yes, a week would be a good start. If we haven't finished everything by then and you don't want to stay longer, we'll look at outpatient treatments." She gestures to the social worker next to her. "Inez will be able to work with you and your family to set those up."

"Okay, I can do that," Blake replies.

Liz draws in her breath. As much as she is relieved that Blake has agreed to accept help, she wonders how a week will solve what has happened to her beautiful boy.

The social worker catches her eye. "We'll make sure we have a solid plan in place before Blake leaves the hospital," she says. "Being home will be good for Blake, and we'll make sure you have all the support you need to help him. And there are support groups specifically for parents of youth with psychotic disorders."

"Thank you," Liz says. A part of her feels that attending the group will mean she and Richard have accepted the worst-case scenario, but another part of her realizes that they have entered a new world with their middle son, one with a changed future and new language.

"It is a very good thing that Blake accepts your role in his treatment and allows us to have meetings with you," Ms. Ramos continues, echoing the nurse's earlier words. "It is hard for families who are completely shut out. The fact that Blake trusts you and seeks your advice is a really good sign."

As she and Richard leave the hospital, Liz thinks about the expert team that Blake has to support him and allows herself to feel a sliver of hope.

What are the treatments for psychosis?

As with other mental illnesses, the treatment options for psychosis include a variety of approaches, including behavioral interventions, therapy, and medication, though in this case, medication is usually one of the first treatment recommendations.

Medications

The single most effective treatment for children with psychotic disorders is antipsychotic medications, of which there are typical antipsychotics (discovered and brought to market between the 1950s and 1970s) and atypical antipsychotics (developed more recently). Although there are some differences between the two classes of drugs, recent research suggests that these differences don't have a significant impact on their effectiveness, only that the newer drugs may have a decreased risk of side effects.[31, 32] Both classes of drugs target the dopamine (a neurotransmitter involved in movement, motivation, and our experience of pleasure and reward) and/or serotonin networks in the brain, which act as signaling pathways between different regions of the brain. The drugs appear to mitigate any disturbances in these networks that contribute to brain cells communicating in atypical ways and causing symptoms of psychosis.

Of course, even the newer medications do have side effects. All antipsychotic medications can cause muscle spasms, abnormal movements, dry mouth, weight gain, restlessness, and other unpleasant and—in some rare cases—life-threatening adverse effects. But an experienced physician will work with your child to find ways to manage these side effects so that your child can remain on the medication as long as he needs in order to return to a relatively normal life. This can take time. Some patients have to try several antipsychotic medications and experiment with dosages before they find one that works for them. For adolescents who have chronic and long-term symptoms and who struggle with taking medication daily, there are long-acting injections that can be administered every one to three months.

There may also be a new generation of pharmacological interventions on the horizon based on glycine and glutamate, neurotransmitters that make up the N-methyl-D-aspartate (NMDA) receptors in the brain, which play a role in learning and memory. Scientists have recently discovered that impairments to NMDA receptors contribute to psychosis—for example, as happens with anti-NMDA receptor encephalitis, a newly understood diagnosis most popularly written about in Susannah Cahalan's 2012 memoir, *Brain on Fire: My Month of Madness*,[33] and the subject of a recent medical review in *The Lancet Neurology*, one of the United Kingdom's leading medical journals.[34]

Psychotherapies

-> Cognitive Behavior Therapy (CBT)

For adolescents who are experiencing a first episode of psychosis or have schizophrenia,[35] CBT, which we have discussed previously, is quite effective in combination with medication. Depending on their symptoms, it can also be helpful for adolescents who are at risk of psychosis rather than those already experiencing clear-cut symptoms.[36]

-> Cognitive Remediation Therapy (CRT)

This psychological therapy is usually conducted with the help of a computer interface and focuses on improving attention, memory, language, and executive function, all cognitive abilities that can be significantly impaired by psychosis. Cognitive remediation, together with vocational rehabilitation, shows promise especially for children with longer-term psychotic disorders.[37, 38]

Behavioral Interventions

As we've discussed previously, this treatment involves practicing healthy sleep patterns, good nutrition, regular physical activity, structured daily routines, and social interaction. Given its effectiveness for children with chronic bipolar disorder, we believe these interventions will help those with chronic psychotic disorders function better in their daily lives, especially those children whose social development may have been interrupted by the onset of their illness.[39, 40]

Family Support

When families educate themselves about psychotic disorders and involve themselves in treatment, they can help their child achieve a better outcome, and this holds true for both those experiencing a first episode or suffering from a more chronic disorder.[41, 42] We work with families to recognize psychotic symptoms and behaviors so that if they occur—and we don't know if they will or not—the family is prepared and can act swiftly. Helping families to communicate, problem solve, and minimize conflict, especially when it becomes frequent and intense, is also an important part of family work. One of the most dangerous aspects of any psychiatric disorder is lack of insight, where symptoms appear to the person to be real experiences rather than stemming from their illness, so it's important that parents talk to their children about what to do if they become ill again and don't recognize what is happening, and agree on a safety plan.

After Treatment

Once the team has finished the majority of the remaining medical tests and explored other potential symptoms with Blake, Liz, and Richard, Dr. Krishnev confirms Blake's diagnosis and recommends an antipsychotic medication, which Blake agrees to take. After a few days, Liz and Richard find Blake more accessible. He accepts their hugs and asks for his *Harry Potter* books to see if he can focus enough to read. It continues to be a challenge to persuade him to remain in the hospital until the doctors are sure he is responding well to the medication, but Inez, the social worker, helps arrange for a full-day home visit near the end of his inpatient stay. It is wonderful to have him there but also strange. Liz can tell that Blake feels tentative around Grant and Meghan, his brother and sister, and when she asks him to set the table for lunch, he circles around the kitchen island as though not sure where to find the cutlery. She has to stop herself from crying and from simply opening the cutlery drawer for him.

By the time of his discharge meeting, Blake is able to focus and participate in the conversation, make eye contact, and respond promptly to questions posed to him.

"We don't yet know how your symptoms are going to play out, Blake," Dr. Krishnev says frankly, "but you've had an extremely positive response to medication so far. We're going to recommend staying on it for two years, as our most recent research indicates that this is the time period associated with the lowest risk of relapse. We also suggest that you participate in cognitive behavior therapy and a teen support group. The good news is that all of these treatments are available to you as an outpatient. How does that sound?"

Liz watches a slow smile grow on her son's face. Richard's hand tightens on hers. Neither of them can remember the last time they saw Blake smile spontaneously.

"Good," he said. "Really good. I want to get home."

"I'm glad," the psychiatrist says, then talks about gradually building up Blake's exposure to stress. "It's like recovering from a concussion. Your brain has taken quite a bruising, and we need to give it time to heal before you return to your old routine." Dr. Krishnev goes on to recommend that Blake continue to have outpatient treatment meetings with his parents, in addition to his individual treatment. "This will help the three of you to make any challenging decisions together, such as deciding when Blake is ready to return to school and consider college."

Just over a year later, Liz looks across the dinner table at her entire family: Richard, Blake, Grant, and Meghan. Grant raises his glass for a toast.

"To Mom and Dad. On your twenty-fifth anniversary. Congratulations, and here's to many more years together."

Blake and Meghan raise their glasses, grinning. "To Mom and Dad. For hanging in there. Congrats!"

Liz's eyes glisten; she knows Richard is thinking exactly what she is: they have just made it through the toughest eighteen months of their marriage.

Blake has continued to take his antipsychotic medication, although he has made it very clear that he wants to try discontinuing it as soon as possible now that he has been symptom free for almost a year. He's back in school and applying to colleges. Grant and Meghan have been his greatest supporters, making sure their brother is never alone if Richard and Liz are at work, and inviting him out with their friends on weekends.

Liz and Richard have been surprised at how helpful the parent support group has been. They've welcomed other parents' advice on setting boundaries and respecting Blake's privacy. Hearing the other moms and dads talk about their fears has also been comforting. The two of them have educated themselves about the risks their son may face, particularly if his psychosis returns, but their social worker, Inez Ramos, who has been with them every step of the way, has both reminded them that none of these grim outcomes is inevitable and encouraged them to focus on the positive factors they and Blake can control.

"You've built a strong family," she said recently. "If Blake has another break, he has you and his brother and sister to support him through it. He won't be alone. Family support is a significant predictor of outcome for patients with psychotic illnesses, and Blake has that covered."

As Liz looks at her family, she knows that Inez has told them something deep and true about themselves and about Blake's future.

ADHD

A Child in Distress

Fred pulls in to the driveway after his long shift at the hair salon he owns. His eight-year-old son, Henry, will be home from school by now and staying with his next-door neighbor Toni and her daughter, Susan. As he walks next door, he hopes that school went well today and that Henry hasn't gotten another detention or an extra assignment.

For some time now, Fred has been worried about Henry. The boy is distracted and rambunctious at home, and his second-grade teacher, Ms. Anthony, says that he's always running around instead of sitting and reading. He's falling behind in class. Fred tries to read to him every night for thirty minutes and to get him to read, too, but it's difficult. Henry has a lot of trouble sounding out the words, and when he gets frustrated, he gives up and asks to watch TV instead. When Fred tells him no, Henry throws a temper tantrum.

At the last parent-teacher meeting, Ms. Anthony said that Henry was in danger of not passing second grade. She also suggested that he might have ADHD. Fred had heard the term before—he dimly recalled that his brother-in-law had it—and knew that kids with ADHD were fidgety, restless, and had a short attention span. Henry exhibits some of those behaviors, but he is just a young kid. Fred mentioned it to his own mother, Mary—who lives out east—during their weekly phone call, and she told him that it was normal, adding that Fred was rowdy as a boy, too, something that he remembers only vaguely.

Ms. Anthony meant well. She knows Fred is raising Henry alone after his wife, Carole, died of breast cancer seven years ago, and she doesn't want him to blame himself. But Fred just can't fathom Henry suffering from an illness after everything they went through with Carole's treatment. She was diagnosed while pregnant with Henry and bravely postponed aspects of her cancer treatment until the later trimesters of her pregnancy so that it wouldn't affect the fetus's development, but she died just before his first birthday. Fred promised he would do his best to raise Henry, but he feels like he is failing. He wishes he had someone to talk to close by about Henry. His mother is so far away, and without Carole, Fred feels alone. He's lucky he can rely on his neighbor Toni.

"I am sorry I'm a bit late," he says when Toni opens the door. "My last client's appointment took longer than I expected."

Toni smiles. "No trouble. Susan and Henry have been playing video games. I haven't heard a peep from them."

"I'm glad he hasn't been any trouble," Fred replies, then calls out Henry's name. "Time to go!"

Henry is too absorbed in the video game to respond, and Fred has to go right up to him, but his son still doesn't look at him. "Henry, I asked you to put down the game."

"Just one more minute, please, please, please?" Henry replies quickly.

"No, you can play later after dinner and homework," Fred says firmly, but it takes several more attempts to get Henry to pay attention to him. Finally, Fred raises his voice; Henry puts down the game. He runs out the door without picking up his backpack or saying goodbye to Toni and his friend.

Fred rushes behind him, and, at the door, Toni hands him Henry's backpack and mentions, "Ms. Anthony said she'd written something in Henry's home book for you to read."

"Oh, thank you," Fred says, taking the bag. He is grateful for the support that Toni provides by picking up Henry from school while he's at work, but he dreads the teacher's message. It's never good news.

The book is an essential means of communication between Fred and Ms. Anthony. Instead of talking on the phone, which is difficult, given both their schedules, Ms. Anthony shares information about Henry's behavior and academic progress at school, and Fred writes back about anything happening at home, such as Henry's being sick or having a doctor's appointment.

At home, Fred gets a cup of tea and settles down with the home book, but Henry has a burst of energy. He runs around the living room, jumps up on the couch, and pesters his father about watching TV.

"But you haven't finished your homework."

"I know, but I want to watch TV," Henry replies.

Fred remains firm and sits Henry down with his schoolwork, but Henry empties his pencil case instead. As Fred picks up the erasers and pencils and markers rolling across the table, Henry takes the opportunity to slide out of his seat and run circles around him. Fred sighs in defeat.

"All right, just for an hour," he says, and Henry plops down on the floor in front of the TV.

With Henry glued to the screen, Fred is free to flip through the pages of the communication book that he has already read. There are lots of comments about difficult and stubborn behavior, refusing to do schoolwork, interrupting in class, not waiting in line during fire drill. Ms. Anthony always makes a point of saying nice things about Henry when he has been courteous, helped a friend, or done well on a math test, but these comments are few and far between. Fred finally gets to the last page:

"Henry had a particularly difficult day today. He seemed upset the moment he walked into school. He couldn't settle at his desk, and at recess, he hit another boy when that boy wouldn't share a toy from the classroom shelves. Has something been happening at home? Have you been able to get an appointment with the pediatrician?"

Fred rubs his forehead. Yes, something has been happening at home. Carole managed the accounting and hiring at their salon. He hired a replacement, but there have been problems with cash flow, and just recently another stylist quit to go back to school, so Fred has been spending his nights looking over the numbers and his days taking on the extra shifts. The stress of dealing with Henry at school and making sure the salon keeps its doors open is becoming unbearable. Fred is at his wits' end.

He looks up and studies his boy, who is engrossed in the TV, and realizes they both need help. He wants Henry to get a good education, which will help him get work where he doesn't have to worry about money like his father does. Fred picks up the phone and leaves a message on the pediatrician's answering service to make an appointment for his son to be assessed for ADHD.

What is ADHD and what are the warning signs?

In the above vignette, Fred wonders if his son's rambunctious behavior is typical childhood energy or a sign of something else. As parents, it's sometimes hard to know the difference. Many children beg to watch TV instead of doing their homework, but if your child is also having trouble meeting developmental and academic milestones, he or she may have ADHD.

ADHD, or attention deficit/hyperactivity disorder, is a common neurodevelopmental disorder that affects a child's ability to pay attention. About 5 percent to 7 percent of children and teens have ADHD,[1] though it typically arises in the preschool years and lessens over time in many children. It's caused primarily by a delay in the maturation of the brain circuits responsible for attention control, which can lead to hyperactivity.[2] In other words, if a child can't keep his attention on something, he's more likely to run around and be impulsive. Eventually most children develop the ability to pay attention, but those with ADHD lag behind and struggle with this more than others, to the point where their behavior impacts how they function at home, at school, and in the community.

As we saw with Henry in the story above, symptoms of ADHD include difficulty sustaining attention, poor concentration, and being easily distracted and impulsive. A child with ADHD will frequently interrupt others and have trouble sitting still and standing in line. ADHD is also associated with overactivity: running around, jumping on furniture, and constant fidgeting.

In ADHD, at least some of its features develop before the age of seven, so these symptoms double as warning signs. The challenge for parents is to differentiate between normal impulsiveness and distractibility and what is a sign of ADHD. Although many kids will exhibit some of these symptoms at some point, by the time they are five, most non-ADHD children are able to pay attention in a variety of situations (not just watching TV or playing video games) and curtail their impulsiveness (for instance, crossing the road without looking). If you're unsure whether your child may be showing signs of ADHD, compare her development with another child of the same age and sex (an older sibling or another child in the neighborhood). If your child differs significantly in the amount she talks, in her ability to pay attention and to use higher forms of grammar, and in her motor skills, and these delays are interfering with her ability to control and sustain attention in a variety of situations, she may have ADHD. If any of these problems interfere with her ability to keep up with her peers in the classroom or affect her social interactions, then it is time to seek help. It is really once a child is in school that it becomes easier to determine if he or she has ADHD, as the comparisons with other children are more distinct, and the requirement to sit still and pay attention is essential to school success. In our next chapter, on autism, we've included a table of some of the most important milestones to watch out for that might signal a child's falling behind in his or her development.

Given that ADHD is a brain-based disorder, a child with ADHD tends to have other neurodevelopmental disorders, such as speech and language disorders, developmental coordination disorders, and learning disorders such as dyslexia.[3] These conditions are more common in boys than in girls and, like ADHD, manifest during a child's early years.

What are the risk factors for developing the disorder?

Environmental Factors

In general, poverty, adverse childhood events, and trauma do not cause neurodevelopmental disorders, but lack of exposure to reading or lack of cognitive stimulation may bring about delays in learning and language development. That's why it's so important for parents to talk, play, and read to their kids—and the earlier the better, and the more sustained the better.

Biological Factors

Genetics play a key role in developing ADHD and other neurodevelopmental disorders (such as learning disorders, and speech and language delays), as these disorders tend to run in families.[4] So, if you or someone else in your family has ADHD, your child faces a higher risk of having it as well. While we can't change our genes, the encouraging news is that being aware of this family history will help make early recognition possible.

In addition to genetic factors and family history, any risk factor that may delay the maturation of the brain can lead to a neurodevelopmental disorder. This includes smoking and drinking alcohol during pregnancy, premature birth, low birth weight, and infection during the baby's first month.[5, 6] One of these events on its own isn't a huge risk, but as a group, they can have significant impact on whether a child develops ADHD or a learning disorder.

Treatment for certain childhood cancers (such as leukemia or brain tumors) can cause ADHD if the brain is directly affected.[7] Similarly, head injuries where the child is unconscious for some time are also associated with later ADHD.[8] Sleep apnea in children, which we described in our chapter on sleep disorders, can lead to daytime sleepiness that mimics ADHD's short attention span and distractibility.[9] Hunger, anemia, thyroid conditions, lead ingestion, and other medical causes are rarer, but every child suspected of having ADHD should have a physical checkup to rule out these unlikely possible causes.

What can parents do to prevent the disorder?

While some genetic risks are unavoidable, the first line of defense against ADHD is good prenatal care, which involves the whole family. This includes familiar basics such as good nutrition and avoiding smoking (and secondhand smoke) and not drinking alcohol. After your child is born, helping him to avoid head injuries is key, so make sure your child always wears a seat belt while in the car and a helmet when bicycling. These are good general practices, but they can also prevent ADHD. Here are a few other tips:

- Read consistently to your child.
- Play numbers games and other activities that will ready your child for school.
- Make sure that your child eats a good breakfast and gets sufficient dietary iron to prevent anemia.
- Watch out for signs of sleep apnea, such as excessive daytime sleepiness and nighttime snoring.

Know that it is not uncommon for some children (especially boys) to lag behind their peers or siblings in different areas of cognitive and motor development, but don't use this as a reason to explain away slow development. We often hear parents make remarks similar to Fred's mother: "Oh, he's just a boy" or "I was like that as a kid, and look how I turned out!" But if your child's delays persist longer than six months or lead to difficulties adapting to kindergarten or first grade, it is time to talk to your family doctor. If she is concerned, she will refer you to a developmental pediatrician, a child psychologist, or a child psychiatrist, who will assess your child.

The sooner a child is evaluated by a physician or psychologist, the sooner his school can make appropriate accommodations for the child's disability. While there are no treatments to speed up brain maturation, many things can be done to accommodate a child's special needs and give him the best chance to meet those milestones.

Reaching a Diagnosis

One month later, Fred and Henry go to the hospital to meet with Dr. Daniel Holder, a developmental pediatrician to whom their family doctor referred them. Dr. Holder is a tall man who looks to be in his late fifties, and the polka dot bow tie he's wearing makes Fred smile, despite his nerves.

The doctor introduces himself and ushers them into his office, which is full of toys. Fred looks around and sees there's no desk, just a few chairs, including some small ones for kids.

"Mr. Marshall, if it's all right with you, I'd like to start our session by watching Henry play with the toys."

"Of course," Fred replies, but inside he feels like everything is riding on this one thing. He looks at his eight-year-old. "Go ahead, Henry. Do you see a toy you like? You're free to go ahead and play with it."

"Cool," Henry says, and he sits down to play with Legos. Fred breathes a sigh of relief. Henry is quite good at putting things together. But after just a minute or two, Henry loses interest in the Legos, gravitates towards the toy tractors, and begins playing with them instead. Fred hopes they will hold his attention, and he won't start running around the room like he often does at home.

After a few moments, Dr. Holder turns to Fred. "Can you tell me what's been going on with Henry lately?"

He fills him in on Henry's behavior at school and at home. "If I'm being honest, he's had these behaviors for as long as I can remember. I just never suspected that they might be caused by ADHD."

"We'll get to the bottom of this. Can you tell me a bit about Henry's development as a baby?"

Fred begins by telling him about Carole's cancer diagnosis and how she forewent treatment until Henry's birth. Henry was born on time but by C-section, as the progress of the labor was slow. Nevertheless, they were happy that there were no complications in the hospital. Henry was a cranky baby but easy to soothe, and generally he slept well. That first year was tough, heartbreaking. Fred was not around Henry much as Carole underwent cancer treatment, but his mother was able to come out and help him. Henry said "Mama" and "Dada" by six months, added a few other words at about twelve months, but waited until forty-two months to use phrases with a verb, which Fred now knows is later than average, having looked it up on the Internet. Henry was also a little slow to start walking by himself without support. He did this at fifteen months instead of at twelve.

"And how was he as a toddler?"

"He had problems focusing. He was always running around, interrupting me when I was talking to someone. In kindergarten, he had trouble sitting still in circle time and holding a crayon or pencil to write and draw." Fred sighs. "And now he is having difficulty reading."

"Henry's trouble with reading and his slow achievement of milestones might indicate that he has a learning disability," Dr. Holder says. "Children with learning disabilities often show ADHD-like behavior at school, but not at home or in the community. At school, the learning disability can make it difficult for them to pay attention to what is going on in the classroom, so they get fidgety and distracted. Can you tell me if you notice these behaviors in Henry at home and with friends, in addition to what his teachers are reporting at school?"

Fred takes a moment to absorb this. "I think his behavior is consistent everywhere. When we go to the mall, I have to keep a close eye on him, or else he'll run away from me to the toy store or to the electronics store. He loves video games. When he's playing video games, he can be quiet and sit still for at least an hour. When we visit his grandparents out east, he gets so excited, he runs around like a puppy."

"I can imagine." Dr. Holder smiles and looks over at Henry, who is back playing with the Lego. "Does Henry have temper tantrums? Do you find it difficult to get him to follow the rules in the house?"

"Sometimes. He gets frustrated easily and stamps his feet and kicks the furniture when he doesn't get what he wants. Last month, he hit a boy at school when they were fighting over a toy, but he's never been violent before or since."

Dr. Holder asks about Fred and Carole's family history, and Fred tells him that Carole's younger brother was a lot like Henry as a boy and was diagnosed with ADHD.

As Fred is talking, Henry comes over and starts tugging at his father's sleeve. "When can we go home?" he asks, then says to Dr. Holder, beaming, "I like your bow tie."

"We are almost done, Henry," Dr. Holder says. "Actually, we could use your help now." He turns to Fred. "I'm just going to do a few checks. Is that okay, Henry?"

Fred watches as Dr. Holder has Henry walk on a make-believe tight rope, then tests how fast he can twist his wrists and touch his thumb to each finger. After the doctor measures Henry's height, weight, and blood pressure, he asks him to take off his shirt and then looks at his skin and listens to his heart and his lungs. Henry complies, but as soon as Dr. Holder is finished, he begins to run around the room and climb on the chairs. Fred tries to calm him, but Dr. Holder tells him it's okay.

"I don't see anything that might indicate a medical reason for him to have these behaviors, and from what I've seen today and from what you've described, it appears he probably does have ADHD." The doctor hands Fred a couple of pieces of paper. "Just to be sure, I'd like his teacher to fill out a questionnaire, so I can get a comprehensive idea of Henry's behavior in the classroom. I'd like you to fill one out as well."

Fred would be lying if he said he hadn't hoped the doctor would give his son a clean bill of health, but on the other hand, a diagnosis means Henry can get the help he needs. Still, there's one thing that bothers him.

"Did everything that happened in his first year cause this?" Fred asks, reluctant to say this in front of Henry.

"No, Mr. Marshall, it most certainly did not," Dr. Holder says kindly. "The part of Henry's brain that controls his attention hasn't yet developed as much as other boys his age. The family history makes me suspect he inherited some of the genetic variants that make ADHD more probable."

As Fred listens to Dr. Holder, he feels a weight lift off his shoulders. "Thank you."

"We'll know more from the questionnaires, but I suspect Henry may also have a learning disability in reading. This isn't uncommon in kids with ADHD. We can have the school test his reading level to make sure, but even so, there is a lot we can do to help Henry."

"Will he have to go on medication?"

"Not necessarily. If the ADHD is mild, we can sometimes improve things with a few environmental accommodations, like having him sit at the front of the class and structuring his time at home."

Fred looks at Henry now, who is playing with the Lego again. "And he'll get better? I don't want him to struggle with this forever."

"These problems may not go away entirely, but with treatment, we can make sure that these ADHD symptoms do not get in the way of his development and become a barrier to him reaching his potential. About 50 percent of kids with ADHD outgrow the disorder, usually in adolescence. The other half can lead successful, productive lives by learning to live with the disorder."

Just then, Henry runs over to Fred. "Can we go now?" he asks.

Fred looks at Dr. Holder, and he nods. "Yes," he tells his son. For the first time in a long while, Fred feels like he and Henry are getting the answers and the help they need.

What are the treatments for ADHD?

As we saw with Fred and Dr. Holder, the first step in treatment is educating parents on what to expect from a child with ADHD. It's important for Fred to see ADHD as a disability and not something Henry chooses to do. It's not his son's fault that he moves around too much, has a hard time sitting still, and is distractible and impulsive. In fact, these behaviors are to be expected of a child with ADHD, and while treatment can include coping strategies and medication, it also involves schools and parents making accommodations and adjustments to help children succeed.

Positive Parenting

Parents are an essential part of treatment. Parenting a child with ADHD can be frustrating. It's natural to want your child to behave even if that means nagging him to sit still or yelling at him not to do impulsive things. But parenting that results in conflict, anger, blame, and a power struggle will not improve your child's ADHD behavior and may lead to worse behavior in the long run.

Positive parenting focuses on teaching parents techniques to contain disruptive behaviors and to provide positive specific feedback about things their child does well. The key is to avoid escalating conflict, by having a consistent routine, clear but flexible rules and expectations, and remembering not to sweat the small stuff. For example, speaking without anger, frequent use of warnings and short time-outs, and using rewards for good behavior can all make a real difference and, in the long term, may have as great an impact on a child's long-term outcome as medication.[10, 11]

One of the first things we recommend is changing how you talk to your children about their ADHD behavior. For example, be honest with your child and acknowledge that sitting still may be a problem for him.

Try saying, "This may be difficult for you, but I want you to try and not move around," or "Remember, you have to stop and think before you cross the road." Over time, these gentle reminders may help a child to incorporate these behaviors habitually.

Here are some other strategies parents can use to help mitigate these types of behaviors at home:

- Avoid situations that will cause conflict. If going to the mall always causes problems, don't go.
- Use a timer to set an amount of time your child has to sit at the dinner table and set realistic goals that bolster his feelings of success and self-esteem.
- Set up a routine at home so that your child knows how much time she has for TV, video games, homework, dinner, and so on. Once she learns the routine, she'll argue less about schedules.
- Work closely with your child's school to institute accommodations where possible, such as moving your child to the front of the class, asking teachers to take an extra moment to ensure that your child has understood instructions, and reducing distractions. In general, shorter activities and frequent breaks help children with ADHD complete assignments.

If your child also has a learning disorder, such as a reading disability, programs that specialize in phonics can make a difference.[12] Phonics teaches children to spell out words by strengthening their understanding of the written syllables and the sounds those syllables make. Parents can do this on their own when reading with their child, but there are also computer games that focus on phonics. At school, special education consultants (such as speech and language therapists and occupational therapists) can work with your child to support him in reading, handwriting, and any other subjects he may be struggling with. For more information about the resources available to you, see our list at the back of the book.

One of the challenges children with ADHD face is the sense of failure that they experience at home and at school. A treatment plan should help them focus on their strengths and build good relationships. Community activities such as soccer, Cub Scouts, or art clubs can boost self-esteem and teach social skills. Children with ADHD can also benefit from sports that require self-discipline, like karate or dance. Any extra-curricular activity that is fun and supports skill building, even in a small way, is a welcome addition to any treatment regime.

Medication

If these accommodations at home and at school are not enough, we recommend trying stimulant medication, which improves attention span and academic skills (such as reading and math), and decreases distractibility, impulsivity, temper tantrums, stubbornness, and aggression. Medication works for about 70 percent of children with ADHD.[13]

The key is finding the right medication and the right dose for your child, and this can take time. Methylphenidate (brand name, Ritalin, Concerta, Biphentin) has had the best results, but if your child experiences unpleasant side effects, there are alternatives, such as amphetamine salts (Adderall), atomoxetine (Strattera), and guanfacine (Intuniv). Each medication has side effects—most commonly a loss of appetite, difficulty falling asleep, and being weepy. When it comes to dosages, sometimes a long-acting dose in the morning is all a child needs to manage his behavior during and after school, through dinner and homework time; another child, though, may require a second dose after school. If your child is lethargic, her dosage is likely too high, and reducing it almost always eliminates that side effect.

Parents often tell us that they're worried that ADHD medications are addictive, but let us assure you that there is no evidence to support this. In fact, these medications can reduce the risk of substance abuse in teens with ADHD, presumably because the medication helps them do better at school and home.[14] There is a valid concern about these medications being diverted from individuals with established diagnoses of ADHD and used by adolescents and young adults who believe mistakenly that taking, say, Ritalin will assist them with their studies. Therefore it is important for parents to ensure that they know where their children's medications are kept, keep track of whether there appear to be missing doses, and educate their child about the risks of giving or selling her medications to other teens.[15]

There is a lot of misinformation on the Internet about the use of drugs for children with ADHD, such as claims that doctors overprescribe medication because the pharmaceutical industry pays them to do so. While it's true that a small number of physicians are paid consultants for drug companies, this is increasingly uncommon because of the conflicts of interest it creates for the medical community. For doctors who are not paid as consultants by the industry, there is no personal incentive to promote the use of drugs to treat ADHD or any other pediatric mental health disorder. If you have these concerns, ask your doctor whether he or she has been paid by the pharmaceutical industry as a consultant, a speaker, or an advisor. It's an appropriate and legitimate question. But remember, the personal interests of a few physicians don't undo the mounting evidence that stimulant medication works for children with ADHD and is safe.

After Treatment

Fred returns home from work after another long day and heads over to Toni's to pick up Henry.

"Hi, Toni," he says when his neighbor opens the door. "Thanks for picking Henry up today. Is he ready to go?"

"Come on in," Toni says. "He and Susan are finishing up their homework right now."

Fred steps inside and sees Henry sitting at the kitchen table. He lights up when he spots his father. "I'm almost done," he says cheerfully. "Can I play video games when we get home?"

It's been three months since his diagnosis. Since then, Fred has worked with Ms. Anthony, who, after consulting an occupational therapist at the school board, has moved Henry to the front of the classroom and signed him up for a reading club. As a result, his grades have picked up. The medication has helped, too. Fred was hesitant to try it at first, but the accommodations at school and at home weren't making enough of a difference. After some trial and error, they have found the right dosage. Henry now takes one pill of a long-acting stimulant in the morning, and that helps him concentrate at school. When he takes the medication, his appetite decreases, so Fred makes sure he eats healthy foods and gets enough sleep. He doesn't give him the medication on the weekend, and then his appetite returns with intensity. Fred is considering taking Henry off the stimulant for summer vacation as well. Dr. Holder reassures him that they will evaluate the need for the medication every year and decide about the upcoming academic year based on how Henry does off the medication during the summer and the early months of school.

Things at the salon have calmed down, freeing Fred to take a course for parents of children with ADHD. He's picked up a number of techniques, which he practices with Henry at home. Sometimes they work, sometimes they don't. His confidence as a solo parent is increasing. He discussed Henry's diagnosis with his mother and filled her in on all that is happening. She is pleased that she knows about her grandson's diagnosis, so she can be helpful when she sees Henry during the summer. "Carole would be really proud of both of you," Mary had said to Fred during their last phone call.

He had had to wipe his eyes before answering. "Yes, she would."

Now, standing in the doorway, Fred smiles at his son. "Yes, if you've done your homework, you can play video games. Can you get your things ready to go?" he asks.

"Yep," Henry replies obediently.

Fred turns to Toni. "Anything in the communication book?" he asks with genuine interest.

Fred no longer dreads what Ms. Anthony might say. In the last three months, they've communicated back and forth, and she's reported that Henry can pay attention for longer periods of time and that he's not bugging the other kids and interrupting her as much. Lately, she's had only nice things to say about him, which is an enormous relief for Fred.

"Nothing to report!" Toni says. "Things have really improved for Henry, haven't they?"

"They really have. I even took him out to the mall last weekend, and it wasn't a disaster. I mean, he's still Henry, he still gets overexcited about stuff, but I've learned to see which behavior is because of his ADHD and which behavior is his choice. He'll always be a ball of energy, but that's just who he is. And I wouldn't want him any other way."

"I'm glad to hear that," Toni says.

Henry tugs at Fred's arm. "I'm ready now."

They say goodbye to Toni and Susan and walk out the door together.

"So, how was school today?" Fred asks.

Henry begins to tell him—talking a mile a minute—about their project to build a volcano, how it exploded all over Ms. Anthony's desk, and how his friend Jessie's volcano did not work at all.

Autism Spectrum Disorder

A Child in Distress

Celia glances at her thirteen-year-old son, Luc, in the backseat of the car. He's playing games on his cell phone. His hoodie hangs low, covering his eyes, but she can see by the set of his mouth that he's unhappy about this visit to a psychiatrist.

"We're almost there," Celia says, but Luc doesn't look up from his phone. "There's nothing to worry about, I'm sure."

Celia exchanges a worried look with her husband, Mark, as he takes the highway exit towards the hospital. They live far from the clinic and have been waiting for this appointment with Dr. Evan Taylor for months. They hope that he can give them some answers about what's happening with their son.

Luc has always been a shy kid who struggled to make friends. He prefers his own company and likes his own routine, so much so that if something changes, like getting new bedsheets, he becomes irritated. Celia and Mark chalked this up to being part of his personality. At times, they wondered if Luc wanted to have more friends, but he always seemed happiest with a book or playing video games.

From a young age, he was a precocious reader and loved going to the library and taking out books with pictures of dinosaurs. He knew all the different types of dinosaurs and would rhyme off the names of different species at breakfast and dinner. The teachers at school were so pleased with his ability to read that they overlooked his irritability and his lack of interest in playing with other children. He learned to count at an early age and could write out multisyllable words by the time he entered first grade. Celia and Mark thought he might even be gifted.

But when Luc was twelve, he started at a new school where his teachers were less lenient about what they called his "antisocial" behavior. He also became a target for bullies. A couple of boys began calling him names and pushing him around in gym. It became so bad that Luc didn't want to go to school. He happily spent all day on his computer, surfing the Internet, going to bed late, then sleeping in. Celia tried to get him to wake up early so he wouldn't miss school, but Luc just yelled that he wouldn't go. He missed so many days that the principal called. When Mark told him that Luc was being bullied, the principal said he would intervene to ensure it didn't continue. Luc returned to school, but the bullying didn't let up.

Then one day two boys grabbed Luc's knapsack and threw it over the fence into the mud. By the time Luc retrieved it, it was soaking wet and covered in dirt. His homework assignment was ruined. Celia and Mark tried to talk to Luc about what happened, but he shut himself in his room. The next thing they knew, the principal called to say that Luc had uttered a death threat over the Internet to the parents of one of the boys.

Celia shudders now thinking of that email. She still can't believe her son would threaten to hurt anyone. Luc apologized, but the principal suspended him and said he needed to have a mental health assessment before coming back to school. The principal specifically asked about an assessment for ASD.

"Do you know what this is?" Celia asked Mark.

He shook his head. Together they looked it up on the Internet.

"Autism spectrum disorder," Mark read out loud.

"Autism?" Celia said. "What do Luc's problems at school have to do with autism?"

That was five days ago. Luc's pediatrician told them that Luc's actions and subsequent suspension constituted a psychiatric emergency and he referred them to their local hospital's urgent child psychiatry clinic. Now Celia and Mark are on their way to the hospital to meet with the psychiatrist.

Celia studies her son, still engrossed with his phone, and wonders, not for the first time, what is going on inside his head. Is this just a phase they're all going through as a family? Or is Luc suffering from a mental illness? And if so, did they miss the signs? She hopes Dr. Taylor can answer these questions.

What is autism spectrum disorder and its warning signs?

In the vignette above, Celia and Mark are worried that their son's behavior may be a sign of something serious, but they are confused when the school suggests his problem may be autism. As a parent, you may be familiar with the term and have some understanding of what autism looks like. For those parents who don't, like Celia and Mark, we are here to explain what autism is and how it affects your child.

Like ADHD, autism spectrum disorder (ASD, or autism for short) is a neurodevelopmental disorder. It, too, is caused by atypical development of brain circuits that support certain functions. But while the brain networks associated with ADHD impair a child's attention span, the ASD networks impair how a child socializes and communicates, and children develop repetitive, stereotyped behavior rather than more imaginative play. Some examples of repetitive behavior include staring at things, running around in circles, and even stamp collecting or learning about dinosaurs (if carried to an extreme), as we saw with Luc. We don't fully understand yet the relationship between these atypical brain circuits and social-communication and play, but the ongoing research suggests that it is a complex issue.

On occasion, we all have trouble socializing or communicating and may become "obsessed" with certain activities. What makes ASD unique is that these differences appear early on in a child's life and are persistent—it is a lifelong disorder. The outward manifestations may change over time (for example, an intense interest in watching water go down the drain changes to an obsession with the local traffic accident rate), but they are always present, even if the manifestations are subtle, as they often are in girls.

It is important to emphasize that many people with ASD live full, meaningful lives, though they do have challenges. Individuals with ASD have difficulty understanding what other people think and feel or what motivates them, and so it's hard for them to talk about emotions or to understand how people feel in response to a certain situation. Children and teens with ASD struggle to recognize that what they do can have unintended consequences for others.

People with ASD also tend to get stuck on details; they have trouble with abstract thought and metaphors. They are excellent at collecting, systematizing, and grouping facts, details, and tidbits of information, but they have difficulty articulating the big picture and understanding theories, nuance, and subtlety. Their attention span is "sticky," meaning that it's hard for them to shift their attention from the details they are concentrating on to something else. So a child with ASD who struggles with a change in routine isn't deliberately being stubborn and difficult. This rigidity and inflexibility are hard-wired into his brain.

We should note that the term *ASD* covers a variety of disorders on the autism spectrum (Asperger syndrome, for one), but the current practice is to use the umbrella term *ASD*, as all the disorders, more or less, share the same symptoms and warning signs, but to varying degrees.[1] In general, the majority of kids with ASD improve over time, some much faster than others. Those who improve more slowly fall further and further behind their typical peers.[2]

ASD is more common in boys than girls and begins to manifest at around six to twelve months of age. Parents typically become concerned about their child's development between one and a half and three years old, though often a diagnosis is not given until after age four or five. This delay in diagnosis may be due to long wait lists for assessment, a provider's lack of knowledge about the warning signs of ASD, or parental lack of education or reluctance to accept that their child has delays. Some early warning signs in infancy include delayed speech, repeating phrases over and over, and being uncommunicative even to the point of not using gestures, such as pointing, to express one's needs. Sensory defensiveness, such as becoming upset at loud noises and certain smells or textures of clothes, is another key sign that your child may have ASD.[3] Repetitive play can manifest in a few different ways:

- doing the same thing over and over again;
- not playing with objects the way they were meant to be played with; and
- being very interested in sensory experiences such as a spinning toy or watching water going down the drain.

On the next page, we've included a snapshot of the important developmental milestones that typical children achieve.

Skills	By two years	By three years
Motor development	• walks without support by twelve months • scribbles and draws • builds a tower of four blocks	• copies a circle • uses utensils and cups • uses a pencil • dresses with some help
Language skills	• says single meaningful words • has communicative babble • points at desired objects • follows simple requests • puts two words together	• says phrases with a verb • imitates with gestures • communicates with gestures • uses plurals • understands most of what is said
Attention development	• is easily distracted • has a short attention span	• starts to focus • starts to concentrate • can shift attention with an adult's help
Social/ emotional development	• has meaningful eye contact • smiles socially • comes to others for comfort • pays attention to faces • is excited to be with peers	• greets others • shows empathy • shows concern for others • separates easily • has a wide range of emotions • is openly affectionate

By four years	By school age
• copies geometric shapes • draws a person • dresses independently • hops on one foot	• has good balance • runs, skips, jumps • catches a ball • writes his or her name
• can hold a back-and-forth conversation • asks who, what, and why questions • uses future tense • tells stories	• has mostly correct grammar • starts to be able to read • writes letters and numbers • engages easily in conversation
• can focus and refocus • can perform an activity and listen	• can sustain attention • shuts out distraction • can start to sit still • can control impulsivity
• has a special friend • plays group games • plays reciprocally • wants to please • can, for the most part, regulate emotions • agrees, for the most part, to rules	• warms up to strangers • has several friends • shares easily • can regulate emotions • initiates social play • plays imaginatively with peers

If you notice your child falling behind, we recommend getting him or her assessed by a psychiatrist, a psychologist, or a pediatrician. There is evidence that the earlier a child is diagnosed with ASD and can get into treatment, the better the long-term outcome.[4] But it is also true that an intervention at any age can still make a difference. It is never too late to get help.

What are the risk factors for developing autism spectrum disorder?

Genetic Factors

We know a great deal more about ASD today than we did a few decades ago. And although there is still much research to be done, we now know that ASD is caused largely by genetic factors that arise spontaneously in the egg or sperm during formation of the embryo. In other words, at conception, as all the bits of biology that make us human come together, rare, small duplications or deletions of DNA may disrupt the genes located in those stretches of DNA that are important in brain development. These structural changes in DNA account for 5 percent to 15 percent of ASD cases.[5] While there is also evidence from family studies that ASD often runs in families, most often the disorder is due to these spontaneous duplications and deletions of DNA at conception, which technically are genetic, but not passed through families or inherited. Presumably, the cause of the other 85 percent of ASD is also genetic, at least in some part, but we have not figured out the actual mechanism at this point.

Environmental Factors

Our understanding of environmental risk factors is limited. We know that the DNA deletions and duplications we've just mentioned are more common if one's parents are older. Unfortunately, as a result of fraudulent research and an epidemic of misinformation, a significant number of parents have been persuaded that vaccination is a risk factor for ASD, but there is no evidence to prove that this is true. In fact, recent studies continue to *disprove* this link.[6] More likely environmental risk factors include prematurity, maternal illness during pregnancy, lack of folate or certain vitamins during the pregnancy, and maternal ingestion of certain drugs such as anticonvulsants.[7]

What can parents do to prevent autism spectrum disorders?

Given the importance of genetic risk factors, there is little that parents can do to prevent ASD. We don't yet know, for example, if reversing those environmental risk factors we mentioned reduces the incidence of ASD. But there are many things you can do to help your child minimize the challenges that ASD poses for him. Let's return to Celia, Mark, and Luc, and find out how a child with ASD is diagnosed.

Reaching a Diagnosis

Dr. Taylor, the child and adolescent psychiatrist, introduces himself to Celia, Mark, and Luc and invites them into the interview room, which is sparsely furnished with a low table and several chairs. They sit down, but Luc avoids eye contact and plays on his phone.

"Luc, I understand you're here today to talk about what happened last week and to be assessed for ASD," Dr. Taylor begins. "Can you tell me what's prompted this?" When Luc doesn't answer, Dr. Taylor turns to Celia and Mark with expectant eyes.

Taking a deep breath, Celia explains what happened at school: how Luc was being bullied, how he threatened the boy's parents, and how he was suspended. When she's finished, Dr. Taylor looks at Luc, who remains silent, swiping at something on his phone screen.

"This must have been pretty stressful for you, Luc. It's awful getting bullied," he says. "I also understand where the school is coming from. Many have adopted a zero tolerance about threats of violence, which is good, but I'm sorry you had to miss school until you saw me."

Luc offers the smallest of nods in response without looking up.

When Dr. Taylor asks Celia and Mark how Luc was as a baby, Luc dives right back into his phone. At first, Celia feels awkward talking about Luc when he's sitting right there, but then she realizes he's tuned them all out.

She tells Dr. Taylor that Luc met all his milestones, but at around eighteen months, he became increasingly cranky, slept poorly, and was difficult to comfort. He didn't like to eat certain foods and preferred macaroni and cheese for breakfast, lunch, and dinner. He hated wearing pants and preferred baggy sweatpants. "As he got older, we tried play-dates, but he's always been shy and hasn't enjoyed playing with other kids. He began to have a difficult time coping with small changes in his routine. For example, one summer Mark grew a beard while on a camping trip with his friends. When he came home, Luc became inconsolable, crying and screaming for hours on end until Mark shaved the beard off. Only then did he settle down."

"I see," Dr. Taylor says. "And have these behaviors persisted over time?"

Celia turns to Mark, then responds. "Yes, I would say so."

"And what about interests? How would you characterize those?"

"First it was dinosaurs," Mark says.

"Then it was baseball," Celia offers. "Luc loves baseball, but not the game itself—the schedules. I once took Luc to the big city to watch a game, but he spent the whole time poring over the program for dates and statistics.

"Now, he's all about the traffic accident rates in major cities, all around the world."

At this, Luc looks up. "Do you know which city has had the highest number of traffic fatalities in the last decade?"

"No," Dr. Taylor replies. "But maybe we can talk about something else? I'd like to know how you feel about the bullying incident that happened at school. Do you still feel like you want to hurt your classmate's parent?"

When Luc returns to his phone instead of answering, Dr. Taylor asks him to put it down. Luc complies but keeps glancing at the phone.

"Can you answer the question, please?"

Luc doesn't speak for several seconds. "No. I guess I said those things when I was mad. It's just that it's so unfair that I get in trouble when they caused all this in the first place."

Dr. Taylor nods his head in agreement. He asks Luc about his emotions, in particular if he feels sad, miserable, or unhappy.

"Miserable," replies Luc. "But not sad or unhappy."

"Can you tell me the difference?"

Luc just shrugs and is silent.

"How long have you been feeling miserable?"

"For a while now." Luc explains that he's worried about black holes in the universe because a new one could be created at any time, and everyone could be sucked into it. He thinks about this possibility a lot. This anxiety, plus his guilt about being suspended from school, keep him up at night. "I'm not convinced that things at school will get any better," he says. "I wish I could get back to my old self."

"Do you think having a few friends might help you feel better?"

"No, I'm quite happy to be by myself. Although it would be nice to go to movies with a friend now and then."

"Thank you for being so honest and open," Dr. Taylor says. Then he asks if Luc has any questions for him. With a smile, the thirteen-year-old asks if he can pick up his phone again. It's the first time Celia and Mark have seen him smile in ages.

"Maybe in a moment?" Dr. Taylor replies. He turns to all of them. "I think we can all agree that Luc overreacted angrily to the bullying at school, but it is important to remember and appreciate that his reaction was understandable. The other kids were bullying him, he tried to find allies among the teachers, but they didn't understand. So he lashed out. He said things that were very frightening to somebody's parents, but Luc himself may have not understood the implications of what he was saying."

Dr. Taylor goes on to explain that there are many different reasons why an adolescent might overreact, but based on what he's heard today, he thinks Luc is struggling with socialization and communication, and has been for some time. "This is what we call autism spectrum disorder, or ASD."

Celia and Mark look at each other and are silent for a bit. "We never thought about autism, till the school mentioned it, did we?" Mark says, turning to Celia.

"Never, though now it sort of makes sense," Celia replies.

"But Luc, you also said that you're miserable and that this is a new problem. I think that in addition to ASD, you might have become depressed in the last year or so. And this has been making your life even harder. Would you agree?"

"Yeah, that sounds right," Luc says.

Celia is stunned. Autism and depression? It's a lot to take in at one sitting.

"Do kids with ASD often get depressed?" Mark asks.

"Indeed they do," Dr. Taylor says. "About twenty percent of kids with ASD get depressed at some point.[8] Some of the most common reasons for kids with ASD to become depressed are conflicts at school with either teachers or peers and bullying. All this means is that Luc should not be blamed for what happened with that threat, but you can work together to make sure something like it doesn't happen again."

"What do you suggest we do?" Celia asks, ready to solve the problem and move on from here.

"There are lots of things you can do to make Luc's life better and allow him to live with his ASD. One important thing to learn is that you as parents have to advocate for Luc with the school. Call the school and tell them that you have seen a psychiatrist who strongly recommends that Luc come back. It's essential that Luc resume a normal life as much as possible and take part in the social and academic opportunities of school. I will support you with a letter to help convince the school."

"Thank you," Celia says. She feels as if a heavy burden has been lifted off her shoulders and can tell by the way Mark is looking at her that he feels the same way.

Dr. Taylor turns to Luc. "Luc, we'll schedule another meeting soon to go over some of the treatment options that are open to kids with ASD. There are a lot of different things we can do, but it's important to have your input. Things may not get better overnight, but if we are all patient and work together, I am sure that you and your parents will be able to master this challenge." Dr. Taylor smiles. "Now you can pick up your phone."

Luc immediately returns to his phone, but he acknowledges Dr. Taylor's words with a nod.

What are the treatments for autism spectrum disorder?

One of the main challenges for Luc in this story is that the diagnosis came so late, even though there were differences in his development very early on. This isn't unusual. Children with ASD who are more cognitively able and have better language skills are more likely to be diagnosed later. That said, if you think your child may have ASD, it's important to have him assessed by an appropriate health care professional as soon as possible, so that he can receive specialized help from his school and community. Speech and language programs, early child development services, special education services at school, community recreational programs for special needs kids, and more specialized programs for kids with ASD provided by community agencies can all make a real difference in both quality of life and in facilitating gains in socialization and communication. The earlier these services are available to children with ASD, the more that can be done to help them thrive.

When we talk about treatment for ASD, we actually mean intervention and support. Be suspicious of anyone who says they have a cure for ASD. Given that ASD presents in many diverse ways, there is no one universal intervention model. When we diagnose a child with ASD, the first things we consider are his age and cognitive ability because supports that work for preschoolers will not work for children or for adolescents like Luc, and supports needed for the more cognitively disabled are not helpful to those more able. Below we walk you through some of the interventions for children of various ages with ASD.

Applied Behavior Analysis (ABA)

When a child is diagnosed early with ASD, we recommend applied behavior analysis, a therapy where children are prompted to learn more developmentally appropriate social, communication, and play skills.[9] Rewards are an important part of the treatment plan, whether that is in the form of food, favorite activities, or other treats. A key component of ABA is that complex skills and more adaptive behaviors are broken down into their component parts and taught to the child with ASD. For example, if a child's ASD is more severe and she has trouble speaking in full sentences, we break down the sentence into its component parts, get the child to learn each part, and then slowly encourage her to put the pieces together and use a full sentence. When she does, we reward her. The earlier a child receives ABA, the greater her chances of improving social, verbal, and play skills.

For children up to five years of age, we recommend at least twenty hours per week of a form of ABA known as early intensive behavioral intervention, or EIBI. This can be a big-time commitment for parents, but depending on the jurisdiction (state or province), EIBI can take place at home, at school, or in the clinic. As the child grows older, it is important to reduce the number of hours of one-to-one therapy so that he gains independence and practices new skills in the real world.

ABA can take many forms. You may prefer a more direct level of intervention, where your child works with a mental health professional or educator on a one-to-one basis for many hours a week (like EIBI). There are also less intensive and intrusive interventions that can take place in day cares and preschools, where educators use naturally occurring opportunities in these settings to promote social and communication and play skills. It all depends on what your child needs. ABA that focuses on building social skills can help children with ASD overcome some of the challenges they face interacting with others, and ABA that includes vocational training can improve job performance for young adults with ASD.[10]

That said, some children, those with severe ASD, may not respond to even intensive forms of ABA. If a child's symptoms interfere dramatically with his development, and he doesn't show significant improvement in his own speech, in understanding the speech of others, in imaginative play, and in social interaction with the help of treatment by the time of adolescence, it's unlikely that therapy will have a major influence on his further development. When this happens, we focus our resources on improving the child's quality of life, helping him to learn key life skills, achieve independence, and reduce behaviors that are more harmful than helpful.

Interventions for Adolescents

With older children such as Luc, who are cognitively able, the forms of intervention that aim to decrease ASD behaviors are not really helpful. Unless there is a specific circumstance or situation that is causing the child stress or he suffers from another mental illness (like depression), we focus more on quality of life and comorbid conditions such as ADHD, anxiety, and depression, not so much on changing ASD behaviors. For people with ASD, making friends, being able to engage in a conversation, having good family relationships, and experiencing success at school and in community activities are important, and the signs and symptoms of ASD are of lesser concern.[11] In fact, the new movement of neurodiversity celebrates the positive differences that ASD brings to the world.[12] People with ASD have many admirable qualities: they tend not to lie, be deceitful, or cruel, and they are not manipulative or mean. Many have special skills in art or music or have a remarkable ability to stay focused on an activity for a long period of time.

Many adults with ASD do not want to be treated or cured, but they do want to have friends, hobbies, vocations, belong to communities, and be physically healthy without mental health challenges. Social skills training, life skills training, vocational training, and help for mental health challenges are the key ingredients of treatment in adolescence and adulthood.[13]

If your child is experiencing stress, our interventions focus on addressing those issues, whether that's through simple behavior interventions such as good sleep habits and healthy nutrition, or coping strategies— favorite activities or "distractors," like going to the movies or bowling— that lift the child's mood. If a child with ASD is also diagnosed with another mental illness such as anxiety, depression, or ADHD, we recommend treatments for those disorders, including therapy and medication. For example, Luc's anxiety about traffic fatalities and black holes is likely a contributing factor to his depression, so by treating his anxiety, we treat his depression, and thus minimize the negative effects of his ASD. There is good evidence that CBT modified for kids with ASD can do much to reduce levels of anxiety.[14] The medications used to treat ADHD that we covered earlier (i.e., stimulants) are useful in kids with ASD who also have ADHD.[15] Sometimes, second-generation antipsychotics such as risperidone (Risperdal) and aripiprazole (Abilify) are used to treat extreme irritability in ASD.[16] As previously discussed, these latter drugs have significant side effects, particularly if there is a family history of cardiovascular disease or diabetes, so parents should have a full discussion of risks and benefits with their child's physician before starting these meds.

After Treatment

After their appointment with Dr. Taylor, Celia and Mark arranged a meeting with Luc's school to explain what was going on with Luc. When they told the principal that Luc had ASD and was suffering from anxiety and depression, he was eager to come up with a plan. Now that they had some understanding of Luc's challenges, they could provide the help he needed in school. It turned out that there were many resources available to Luc.

Together, his principal and Celia and Mark set up a special meeting with educational specialists to modify Luc's program to accommodate his needs. For example, his teachers were encouraged to use his special interests as a motivating factor to teach from the curriculum. He could be taught science using the physics of black holes as a content vehicle. He could be taught mathematics using the traffic fatality rates in different cities as examples. The school also adopted a zero-tolerance program towards bullying, with class discussions, posters in the hall, and bringing in public speakers. With the reassurance that Luc understood the consequences of his actions and his promise that he would try his best and accept help to contain his anger, the principal allowed him back at school and promoted him to ninth grade, despite his having missed so much of eighth grade.

At home, Mark and Celia organized a schedule that would help Luc get enough sleep and encourage other activities besides playing on his phone and computer, which they moved out of his bedroom and into the TV room so they could monitor his use. They made sure the schedule was detailed, as they knew now that having a routine calmed him and left no room for unanticipated changes that might cause anxiety. If changes cropped up, they gave him ample warning whenever possible and encouraged him to use his new coping strategies to moderate his anxiety. After a rocky start, Luc adapted to the schedule and fell into a comfortable routine. Over time, there was less friction at home and at school, and Luc's anxiety and depression lessened.

He even developed a friendship with a boy at school who was also on the autism spectrum. Both were interested in outer space, but his friend didn't worry about black holes, which Luc still did. Nevertheless, Celia was able to see how Luc could use his interest in space to structure a friendship with another child. Mark and her both thought there was a real bond there, even if it focused on a single topic.

"Who's to say this relationship is any less real than the friendships that typical kids develop?" Celia said.

One day Celia noticed Luc was spending more time on the computer than allotted on the schedule. When she walked over to see what he was doing, Luc explained that he was talking to some really cool people on the Internet.

"They are 'Aspies,'" he said with a smile, staring at the screen.

"Aspies?" Celia echoed. "Who or what are Aspies?"

"There is this chat room with other people who have Asperger syndrome. And it's really cool. I'm learning so many neat things about people like me! Never knew it."

Celia smiled. "That's very nice." Then she reminded him that it was time for dinner, but inside, she was overjoyed that Luc had found a new community.

At a checkup with Dr. Taylor a year later, Luc tells him how things have improved. He no longer feels miserable or anxious. He still does not meet the doctor's eyes, but he is not fixated on his phone.

"I'm glad to hear it," Dr. Taylor says. He turns to Celia and Mark. "And what about you?"

Celia smiles at her son. "Luc's passion for learning and reading were always things we loved about him. We now know that part of that comes from his ASD, and so long as he's healthy and happy, we continue to celebrate those things. We realize he'll have challenges, but now we know what we can do to help."

"Good. And all that changed with a diagnosis. As soon as we knew what was going on with Luc, we could help him alleviate distress. It's not so much the ASD that is a problem for Luc, it's the challenges of living with it in our world. Where we can, we'll help the world accommodate Luc, and on occasion, we'll help Luc accommodate the world. He has enormous potential to be happy and to thrive. Other challenges will crop up in the years to come, and we will meet each one head on." Dr. Taylor turns to Luc. "What do you think of that, Luc?"

"It sounds like a clear and reasonable plan," Luc responds.

"Clear and reasonable," Celia repeats to Mark on the way home. Never has she been more relieved by her son's words.

Conclusion

As we said in our introduction, *Start Here* is just that, a starting point. We hope that our overview of these child and adolescent mental health issues has answered some of the questions you may have had but also provided you with a way forward if you are concerned that your child has a specific mental health problem. In that case, we encourage you to learn more by checking out our resources section, speaking to your child's doctor, and doing your own research as well. Whether or not you need to navigate the mental health system, we hope we've assuaged some of your worries and given you tools to help your child. We emphasize the word *help*—not *fix*, not *cure*, not *solve*—as mental health is a continuum. Wellness doesn't happen overnight. It's trial and error. Be patient, open, and understanding with both your child and yourself. And remember: getting angry or blaming yourself or your child is never productive.

The best thing you can do to support your child's physical and mental health is to provide him or her with a structure that promotes healthy sleep, good nutrition, enough physical activity, appropriate screen time use, and positive, caring relationships, from an early age. And learn about risk factors, especially family history and childhood experiences that may put your child at risk. While there is no guarantee that your child will not develop a mental illness, being aware of the risks and providing your child with support may prevent (and certainly mitigate) these factors from causing future mental illness.

Of all the challenges we've discussed in our book, one of the most important warning signs is drastic changes in your child's behavior or ability to function successfully at school and with family and friends. Again, we urge you not to write off these changes as a phase, but to talk to your child and try to find out what is going on. It can be an awkward conversation, but enduring some discomfort to put your worries to rest or to get your child early help is well worth it.

Your child's school can be a great support system. We know parents—and children—are sometimes wary of sharing mental health information with schools, and we understand this, but it's possible to gather useful information while placing boundaries on what you decide to share with them. As we saw in our vignettes, a child's teachers can help parents determine whether their child is deviating from academic, behavioral, or social expectations and if he or she requires a developmental or mental health assessment. Schools can also direct parents to educational resources.

If you and your child seek professional help, we recommend coming to your appointment prepared with a point-form description of changes in your child's behavior, academic performance, and, if relevant, his or her difficulties achieving certain milestones. It doesn't need to be a tome; you want your child's clinician to be able to digest the information efficiently, but noting timelines and interventions that worked for a while or made things worse is very helpful. This ensures your child's health care provider has a full picture right from the start.

As our children grow up, they become more independent and self-sufficient. While it's important to respect their privacy, talk to your children about what can and cannot be kept private at different stages of their lives. For example, younger children should be reminded to share with adults any experiences of abuse and bullying. And while this may be controversial, we recommend that parents have access to all their child's social media accounts at least up until high school. Middle school and high school students should be encouraged to share any concerns about their friends' behavior and mental health, including issues of safety. All of these conversations are good to have periodically, especially if you and your child need to navigate the mental health system together.

And, of course, the tasks of parenting don't cease when your child becomes an adult in the eyes of the law and society. When your child has mental health issues, the transition to emerging adulthood can be particularly challenging because he may not want you to be involved in his medical care. If that's the case, his health care providers must respect his decision. You may wonder how to support a legal adult who relies on you financially without undermining his or her independence and self-reliance. Or what the boundary is between seeming interested and being intrusive after a child has moved out of the family home. For a parent of a child who has or is struggling with a mental illness, these questions can sometimes have life-or-death consequences. There are no easy answers for how to handle these situations, but being open and respectful with your child while raising concerns honestly is always important.

We know that it is hard to take a step back, especially when a parent has spent a whole lifetime advocating for a child with a developmental or mental health problem, but there *are* ways to navigate these challenges so that a previously or currently unwell child can take more responsibility for her health care and life tasks, and parents can continue to play a role, albeit less involved and directive. Negotiating with your child and having her provide permission to her health care providers about what can and cannot be shared with you as parents prior to her achieving an age of majority is key. Think about what you would have been comfortable sharing with your parents, while factoring in what may be different in your relationship with your child. Don't expect to know everything, but figure out together what may be preventative knowledge for you to have. For example, if your child's mental health starts to affect his education or employment, that may be a marker for when you will become more involved. Again, you do not need to know every detail, just that your child may need more support.

Some parents have told us that accepting the natural and legal boundaries that exist for adults in our health care system has actually been the hardest aspect of dealing with their child's illness. However, it can also be an opportunity—to renegotiate your support for your child and to demonstrate confidence in your ability to work together collaboratively while respecting his or her privacy.

We understand that the isolation experienced by parents coping with a child's mental illness can be as great or even more of a disability than the illness itself. We hope that by shedding light on the frequency and nature of children's mental illness—and the many treatment options available—we have helped destigmatize mental illness and made you feel less alone. Yes, you may sense judgment from others and feel exhausted and powerless at times. Your own mental health may suffer as you try to help your child. But remember, you are not alone. There is help for you, too. Before we close, we want to remind you who can help *you*.

We urge you to resist the shame that many parents still associate with having a child with a mental health disorder that may be holding you back from reaching out to those close to home: your coparent (if relevant), your family, your friends, your own doctor or other health professionals, and, perhaps as we have just discussed, your child's school. In all these cases, with the possible exception of your coparent and health care providers, it is important to negotiate and be honest with your child about what can be shared and what will remain private. Remember that your coparent—whether you are together or apart—has a shared responsibility for your child's well-being, and can be a primary support to both your child and to you (unless in the rare instance they themselves are unstable or a source of significant stress). Your own and your child's health care providers all have a legal responsibility to maintain both your privacy, and while the latter cannot disclose your child's private health care information to you except in the case of emergency, they are able to take information from you. If they recommend you seek support for yourself from a mental health professional, anything you share with that individual remains confidential, unless you or someone else is at immediate risk. Consider joining a parents' support group, even if you feel too tired to go initially. Parent after parent has told us that knowing that other moms and dads are facing similar challenges has been a life saver for them. Find out about community programs—after-school programs, summer camps, mentoring initiatives—designed for children with mental health challenges and their families. By sharing your experiences and concerns, you are not only helping yourself and your child, you are helping other parents who are struggling with their internalized stigma and self-blame.

It is an impossible burden for parents to shoulder sole responsibility for the mental health of their children. We all share it. To borrow a familiar phrase, "It takes a village." On the following page we've listed some essential community resources that help parents support their children's mental health. Unfortunately, they do not exist everywhere and can be at risk in times of public financial constraint, but we urge all parents and health care professionals to advocate for these supports. For parents who are in the midst of crisis, your first job is to look after your child, yourselves, and your families, but once your child has reached a safer place, we encourage you to spread the word about programs that either helped you or that you wish had been available to you.

- Early intervention and education programs for vulnerable children and families;
- Free breakfast and lunch programs for children coming from impoverished homes;
- Safe outdoor environments that promote children's physical activity;
- A mental health system that provides timely affordable access to proven therapies, not just medication;
- Universal child care;
- After-school programs, particularly for vulnerable youth;
- Mental health resources in schools;
- Mental health professionals embedded in family health teams;
- Policies and legislation aimed at preventing or mitigating adverse childhood experiences (ACES) such as abuse and neglect;
- A well-resourced, culturally safe, expert child protection system that can maintain safety for a child while supporting a relationship with parents who require their own mental health treatment for addiction, illness, or their own experience of trauma;
- Legislation and economic support for parents who need to take time away from their work to care for a mentally ill child;
- Advocacy for Indigenous communities—both rural and urban—through policies and funding opportunities that have been associated with improved health and mental health outcomes for children and youth.

Finally, we want to remind you of our book's most important message: Don't look away from your child's distress. Don't try and comfort him too quickly. Insist on spending time with your child even if he resists, but meet him halfway by offering to do something he is interested in. Be proactive. Risk overreacting. Ask difficult, awkward questions. Learn about the behaviors she is exhibiting that worry you and make sure you rely on good sources that refer to science and well-researched evidence. Talk to your own support network and to health professionals whom you trust about your concerns and get their advice and help.

While we understand every parent's fear of facing the possibility that something is truly wrong with your child's mental health, we also know that the consequences of looking away can be tragic. Deep down, your child wants and needs your help. He's counting on you to obtain for him the care he needs. We hope this book reassures you that you are indeed capable of making a positive impact on your child's mental health. We have provided the information, resources, and supports; we know that you will bring the love, courage, persistence, and honesty required to help you, your child, and your family find your way forward to a better place.

Authors' Note

While we have drawn on our shared clinical experiences to create the book's fictional vignettes, which illustrate specific disorders and the challenges they raise for families, none of the children and adolescents described in them are actual patients, nor are their families based on real individuals. Any resemblance to any child, adolescent, parent, family, or individual we have seen in our careers is entirely coincidental. While we recognize the unique power of actual patients and families to fight stigma by sharing their real-life experiences, their stories are not ours to tell, especially given that our patients are minors who may feel differently about their privacy as they grow older.

A note on our sources. We would like to address directly the issue of evidence. It is essential for parents—and children and teens—to be able to distinguish between facts and evidence derived from rigorously and painstakingly conducted research that has been ethically and scientifically reviewed, and an individual's opinion and advertising. In *Start Here*, we have referenced only evidence derived from academic, peer-reviewed research and/or supported by government or appropriately credentialed health care institutions. Where we have presented our own opinions, based on our shared clinical experience, we have explicitly said so. We are grateful to our expert colleagues who have reviewed specific chapters to ensure we have met our own standard. (See "Acknowledgements.") Any errors that slipped through or were inadvertently added after their review are ours alone.

For this reason, we have not discussed a number of emerging treatments that have promising—and rigorously conducted—research to support their use in adults and may become relevant to children's mental health in the future: brain stimulation therapies for mood disorders, psychotic disorders, OCD, and eating disorders that have not responded to conventional treatments; ketamine for treatment-resistant depression; and the use of anti-inflammatory agents or stem cells for psychiatric disorders. Until these have a stronger evidence base to support their safe and effective use in children and adolescents, we will leave their discussion to future books.

We would also like to apologize in advance for any resources we've provided here that become no longer available between the book's writing and readers' accessing. It is the gift and burden of citing easily accessible (and easily de-accessible) online resources.

Acknowledgements

All books require thank-yous, and ours is no exception. First and most important, we need to thank our patients and their families for their patience, trust, and willingness to educate us on their concerns and questions. It is the decades of trying to respond to the latter that led to our desire to write this book, as we recognized that the vast majority of the questions and anxieties raised were consistent among families, even when the disorders their children faced differed.

We thank our psychiatrist and health care colleagues who help us care for patients by sharing their expertise and academic knowledge with us, and for their willingness to cover clinically for us to ensure we get the time for academic projects such as this book. We recognize that after this book, we owe them a significant debt!

We specifically want to thank our expert readers who generously read our chapters to ensure that nothing we convey is misleading or out of touch with current scientific evidence: Dr. Suneeta Monga for anxiety disorders; Drs. Karen Leslie and Trisha Tulloch for substance use disorders; Dr. Seena Grewal for eating disorders; Dr. Shelly Weiss for sleep disorders; Drs. Daphne Korczak and Benjamin Goldstein for mood disorders and suicidality; Dr. Aristotle Voineskos for psychosis; and Nurse

Practitioner Cathy Maser for sexual orientation and gender identity as a potential risk factor for mental health concerns.

An additional thank-you to our British colleague Dr. Isobel Heyman at London's Great Ormond Street Hospital for generously sharing her time and thoughts about child and adolescent psychiatry trends in the United Kingdom.

We were lucky enough to have exceptional help finding relevant resources and background material: thank you to both Kathryn Semogas, who ensured that our references, glossary, and resource materials were in tip-top shape, and Karissa Holyer, who will undoubtedly support children's mental health in her future medical career.

Thank you to Shanique Edwards, Hiba Michael, Olga Serebrennik, and Olesya Zaremba, who tirelessly protected us to give us a day a week free from our academic, clinical, and administrative obligations in order to write.

Thank you to our hospitals, The Hospital for Sick Children and the Centre for Addiction and Mental Health, and to our academic home, the Department of Psychiatry and Faculty of Medicine at the University of Toronto, for supporting our intellectual work. While our clinical work always feels the most urgent, having opportunities to engage in scholarship, teaching, research, and advocacy to ensure that our field continues to move forward is a gift.

Thank you to Jennifer Glossop, who helped us to conceptualize initially what parents want and need to know, and who encouraged us to turn a desire to help into a book proposal.

Both of us are grateful beyond words to our editors at Simon & Schuster: Sarah St. Pierre and Nita Pronovost. Sarah personifies the editor as both therapist and skilled creator of readable books, encouraging us, challenging us, and nudging us to make sure *Start Here* is a book that will actually help parents rather than collect dust in a health sciences library. Nita, who oversaw this project, cut through our medical tendency to be overinclusive and focused us on our core messages.

Thank you to Adria Iwasutiak, Felicia Quon, Catherine Whiteside, Alexandra Boelsterli, Paul Barker, Aneeka Sihra, and the entire team at S&S for ensuring our book made it into bookstores and sales catalogues and found an audience. Special thanks to Philip Bashe, our copy editor, whose assiduous edits improved the book remarkably.

Thank you to Kevin Hanson, our publisher, for his determination to bring books on mental health written by experts to the public. He is both a champion and an advocate.

Thank you to Michael Levine and the team at WCA for their support and guidance on not only brainstorming ideas but on all matters contractual.

Thank you to all our friends who shared with us what they would want as parents from a book on children's mental health. They encouraged us to be honest about the real risks and challenges faced by families with children who have mental health issues, while instilling hope about the help that is available to them.

And finally, but never least, to our own families, who put up with our distractedness and who generously gave us leaves from household chores while the book was being written. More important, their enduring love reminds us daily of what gets families through the toughest times.

Resources

Who Does What in Children's Mental Health?

Profession	Role
Special education experts	These professionals are usually trained teachers who have additional training in supporting children with special needs, such as diagnosed learning disorders and developmental and attention challenges. They contribute to independent educational plans, which involve accommodations and additional academic supports to ensure these children's educational success.
Child psychologists	These are professionals with master's degrees or PhDs who may provide in-depth educational assessments and therapy. Unlike many nonphysician health care professionals, they are able to provide mental health diagnoses.
Child and youth workers (sometimes called child and youth counsellors)	Graduates of college programs who have training in how to work with children and youth. They sometimes staff resource classrooms, youth mental health centers, and hospitals. They can also work in private practice.

Profession	Role
Child therapists	This simply refers to a therapist who has extra training in working with children. It is important to ask what that training is and whether the therapist is a member of a registered professional association, such as the Canadian Association for Play Therapy, or the American Association of Child and Adolescent Psychiatry. There are also province- and state-specific associations.
Art therapists	Therapists who have training in working with art as a means of therapeutic expression and connection. In addition to asking about an art therapist's credentials, it is important to know if he or she has had additional training and experience working with children and adolescents.
Behavioral specialists	Professionals with training in using behavioral approaches based on learning theories to help a child to achieve change. For example, a therapist who is trained in applied behavior analysis (ABA), will have skills and training specific to working with children with autism spectrum disorders.
Occupational therapists	Health care professionals who have expertise in helping unwell or disabled individuals to develop or recover skills required for daily living.
Developmental pediatricians	Medical doctors and pediatricians who specialize in the diagnosis and treatment of children with developmental delays or variations, and behavioral challenges. Like child and adolescent psychiatrists (see below), these doctors can diagnose, prescribe medications, and potentially (although less commonly) conduct emergency assessments and hospitalize children, if needed, if they work in or are associated with a hospital.

Profession	Role
Child and adolescent psychiatrists	Medical doctors who complete extra training in adult and then child and adolescent psychiatry, and have additional certification in the diagnosis and treatment of childhood psychiatric disorders. They can diagnose, prescribe medications (including psychiatric drugs), conduct emergency assessments, and hospitalize children.

Where Can I Get Help for My Child?

Place	Help
Online apps	There is a proliferation of online mental health apps for children and young people. Some are designed and researched by universities and government; others are simply someone's bright idea or entrepreneurial project. We recommend asking your child what apps he or she is using and ensuring they are supported by an institution or individual with appropriate training and credentials.
Support groups	These are not treatment, which is important to understand, but may provide invaluable support to a struggling child or adolescent or to parents who want to understand how they can help. Support groups are sometimes but not always facilitated by a trained mental health professional.
Walk-in mental health centers	Drop-in centers where a child or adolescent can be seen on a same-day basis for a mental health appointment. Some mental health centers use a drop-in format as the intake for their long-term treatments for children and adolescents who need more than the occasional drop-in appointment.

Place	Help
Children's mental health centers or CMHCs (specific to Canada), or other publicly funded agencies to support children's mental health	Publicly funded agencies that provide children and adolescents with evidence-based psychotherapies, meaning therapies supported by scientific studies. Some will have a child and adolescent psychiatrist consultant, others do not. Usually these centers offer individual, group, and family therapy, mental health education, and support groups. We strongly encourage families to use their local CMHCs when they are available, as an easily accessible location can make a huge difference in minimizing the disruption inherent in attending regular appointments for both the child (particularly with regard to missing school) and for family members. These may be funded nationally, or by provincial, state, or municipal governments.
Therapists in private practice	Individuals from a variety of professional backgrounds who work alone or with a few colleagues in a community office and charge fees (sometimes covered by health insurance plans) for individual and/or family therapy. Private therapists tend to have shorter waiting lists and more flexibility in the timing of appointments, but cost is a drawback for most families.
Day or inpatient treatment	May refer to foster care, residential treatment, wilderness camps/therapeutic boarding schools. These are all more intensive treatment options for when a child cannot be treated safely or effectively as an outpatient. For each place to offer mental health treatment, they need to have trained staff, appropriate mental health support, and oversight.
Crisis lines	Phone lines that children and adolescents can call or text can literally be a lifeline, allowing children to speak anonymously if they wish to communicate with a volunteer who is trained to help them in a crisis. Children will speak to a different volunteer whenever they call, so there is no continuity available. Your child's communication with the crisis line is confidential, but in situations where the child is in immediate danger, volunteers can alert 911.

Additional Resources

General Resources for Parents, Families, and Children

About Kids Health is a health education website for children, youth, and their caregivers, developed by Toronto's Hospital for Sick Children. Their online resource hub has information on:

- Age-Specific Issues: https://www.aboutkidshealth.ca/hcp
- Mental Health: https://www.aboutkidshealth.ca/mentalhealth
- Parenting Learning Hubs: https://www.aboutkidshealth.ca/parenting

For a complete listing of information on all the mental health challenges we've discussed in this book, go to https://www.aboutkidshealth.ca/>Menu />Health A-Z. Additional reading materials and resources on each topic are included in the resource section.

Beyond Blue is an Australian nonprofit initiative, funded in part by government, that provides a framework for understanding the spectrum of mental health and the difference between mental health and mental health conditions: https://beyou.edu.au/resources/mental-health-continuum.

Big White Wall is an online mental health support community for individuals who are sixteen years old and over. It is available 24 hours a day, 7 days a week and is monitored by trained "Wall Guides" who help users navigate the site and ensure it is safe and anonymous. Members help and support one another, and also have access to guided online courses and self-help tools. In the United Kingdom, it's available here: https://www.bigwhitewall.co.uk/ and in Ontario, Canada, through the Ontario Telemedicine Network (OTN) here: https://www.bigwhitewall.ca/v2/Home.aspx.

Caring for Kids is a website developed by the Canadian Paediatric Society—the voice of more than 3,300 Canadian pediatricians—that provides expert guidance and strategies from Canada's pediatricians about how to foster good mental health: https://www.caringforkids.cps.ca/handouts/mental_health.

Centre for Addiction and Mental Health (CAMH) is Canada's largest mental health teaching hospital. See their suggestions for strategies for fostering resilience in children and teens here: https://www.camh.ca/en/health-info/guides-and-publications/raising-resilient-children.

Good2Talk is a free, confidential, twenty-four-hour helpline that provides support to post–secondary school students ages seventeen to twenty-five in Ontario, including resources and information, referrals to services on campus and in the community, and anonymous single-session counselling over the phone in English and French. Good2Talk is a partnership between ConnexOntario, Kids Help Phone, Ontario 211, and the Ontario Centre of Excellence for Child and Youth Mental Health and is funded by Ontario's Ministry of Advanced Education and Skills: https://good2talk.ca/.

Healthline is a consumer health information website dedicated to making health and wellness resources accessible through their site, newsletters, apps, podcasts, and communities. They cover everything from ADHD to depression: https://healthline.com.

Jack.org is a Canadian charitable organization working to train and empower young people to "understand how to take care of their own mental health and look out for each other." Their resources include a "Mental Health 101" primer, and guidance on where to find help: https://jack.org/Resources/Learn.

mindyourmind is a government of Ontario–sponsored site that provides interactive online tools for youth to build capacity and resilience and is developed in partnership with youth: https://mindyourmind.ca/tools.

MQ: Transforming Mental Health, a charitable research organization in the United Kingdom, has an informative "News & Blog" section on their website that includes individual stories, a podcast, and updates on mental health research: https://www.mqmentalhealth.org/news-blog/category/science-and-research.

Orygen, Australia's National Centre for Youth Mental Health, offers resources for young people and their families including toolkits and research bulletins: https://www.orygen.org.au/Education-Training/Resources-Training/Resources, and webinars for health professionals and community workers, which may also be of interest to parents and caregivers: https://www.orygen.org.au/Education-Training/Resources-Training/Webinars.

The Offord Centre for Child Studies, a multidisciplinary research institute focused on improving the lives, health, and development of children and youth, publishes "knowledge pamphlets" on a range of topics. These resources are available online and have been translated into several languages including Inuinnaqtun and Inuktitut: https://offordcentre.com/research/knowledge/.

YOUNGMINDS.org is a British charity focused on youth mental health. Their website includes toolkits and guides on mental health challenges for parents: https://youngminds.org.uk/find-help/for-parents/.

Anxiety Disorders

Anxiety Canada is a charitable organization that provides education and tools for individuals suffering from anxiety, including the MindShift CBT app: https://anxietycanada.com/.

Caring for Kids has information on SSRI use in treating depression and anxiety here: https://www.caringforkids.cps.ca/handouts/using_ssris_to_treat_depression_and_anxiety_in_children_and_youth.

Substance Use Disorders

American Academy of Pediatrics (AAP) is an organization of 67,000 pediatricians committed to the optimal well-being of children and youth. See their suggested steps that parents can take to prevent drug use here: https://patiented.solutions.aap.org/handout.aspx?gbosid=166256. For specific information on tobacco, visit here: https://www.healthychildren.org/English/health-issues/conditions/tobacco/Pages/default.aspx.

CAMH has educational information on addiction: https://www.camh.ca/en/health-info/mental-illness-and-addiction-index/addiction.

"Counseling Parents and Teens About Marijuana Use in the Era of Legalization of Marijuana" by Sheryl A. Ryan and Seth D. Ammerman includes key takeaways for parents: https://pediatrics.aappublications.org/content/139/3/e20164069.

The Government of Canada has an online listing of the supports for problematic substance use available in Canadian provinces and territories, including 24 helplines for youth and adults and links to organizations: https://www.canada.ca/en/health-canada/services/substance-use/get-help/get-help-problematic-substance-use.html.

For information about e-cigarettes, here is a tip sheet to help parents talk to their teens about the health risks associated with vaping: https://www.canada.ca/content/dam/themes/health/publications/healthy-living/vaping-mechanics-infographic/Parent%20tip%20sheet_web_Final_EN.pdf.

U.S. Government National Institute on Drug Abuse for Teens provides facts and tools for teens, parents, and teachers: https://teens.drugabuse.gov/teens.

Eating Disorders

Center for Young Women's Health at Boston Children's Hospital has developed guides for parents that dispel common myths about eating disorders and help parents prepare their child for a medical evaluation: https://youngwomenshealth.org /eating-disorders-for-parents-all-guides/.

F.E.A.S.T. is an international organization that offers help to parents of individuals with eating disorders, including a global support community with a presence in seventy countries: https://www.feast-ed.org/.

National Eating Disorder Information Centre (NEDIC) is a charitable organization administered by the University Health Network and is based at the Toronto General Hospital. NEDIC provides support, resources, and referrals to Canadians through a toll-free helpline and online instant messaging: https://nedic.ca/.

BC Children's Kelty Mental Health Resource Centre has created a video series called "Eating Disorders Meal Support: Helpful Approaches for Families," which features real-life stories from youth and parents. The series is available on their YouTube channel: www.youtube.com/keltymentalhealth.

Sleep Disorders

American Academy of Sleep Medicine publishes patient education materials and a Sleep Health & Wellness Blog: http://sleepeducation.org/.

Canadian Sleep Society, a professional association of researchers and clinicians that supports research and promotes public education, has a wide range of information on their website as well as suggestions on books and publications that provide in-depth insight into sleep disorders and how to manage them: https:// css-scs.ca/.

Royal College of Psychiatrists in the United Kingdom provides guidance for parents and caregivers on sleep problems in childhood and adolescence: https://www .rcpsych.ac.uk/healthadvice/parentsandyoungpeople/parentscarers/sleepprob lems.asp.

The Sleep Fairy by Janie Peterson and Macy Peterson (2003) is a children's book that teaches children to stay in their own beds through the night.

Depression, Trauma, and Suicidal Thoughts

Children's Hospital of Eastern Ontario (CHEO) offers tips for parents to help children and youth who are feeling suicidal, including a suicide safety plan: https://www.cheo.on.ca/en/resources-and-support/suicide.aspx#Fact-sheets.

The American Academy of Pediatrics (AAP) provides tips to help parents support teens experiencing depression. "Adolescent Depression: What Parents Can Do to Help" is available here: https://www.healthychildren.org/English/health-issues/conditions/emotional-problems/Pages/Childhood-Depression-What-Parents-Can-Do-To-Help.aspx.

The Cundill Centre for Child and Youth Mental Health at CAMH is a research center that generates new knowledge about child and youth depression and shares that knowledge with families and health care practitioners around the world. Their website features resources for parents and youth about treating depression and tools for clinical care: https://www.camh.ca/en/science-and-research/institutes-and-centres/cundill-centre-for-child-and-youth-depression.

The Marjorie E. Korff PACT Program at Massachusetts General Hospital has published "Community Crises and Disasters: A Parent's Guide to Talking to Children of All Ages," a useful guide for parents on topics such as managing media use, self-care, and tips for talking to children about a disaster or crisis: https://www.mghpact.org/assets/media/documents/MGH%20PACT%20Guide%20(Talking).pdf.

WE MATTER is an Indigenous and youth-led nonprofit organization in Canada that supports Indigenous youth who are dealing with addiction, depression, sadness, and pain. Their multimedia campaign features messages from role models and allies. Toolkits for youth, teachers, and community workers are available through their website, which also includes information on where to get help: https://wemattercampaign.org.

Psychosis

CAMH's "First Episode Psychosis: An Information Guide" by Sarah Bromley, Monica Choi, and Sabiha Faruqui provides information on types and stages of psychosis, treatment, family involvement, and the process of recovery: https://www.camh.ca/-/media/files/guides-and-publications/first-episode-psychosis-guide-en.pdf?la=en&hash=E217B7A693F6AE0E4242A6535F922C50A1E24F78.

Mayo Clinic has comprehensive information on symptoms, diagnosis, and treat-

ment of schizophrenia available on their website here: https://www.mayoclinic
.org/diseases-conditions/childhood-schizophrenia/symptoms-causes/syc-20
354483.

Mind, a mental health charity in the United Kingdom, shares real-life stories of
youth and adults living with psychosis on their website and podcast, as well as
tools and strategies for self-care: https://www.mind.org.uk/information-support
/types-of-mental-health-problems/psychosis/#.XYJ_qSV7kWo.

ADHD

"Caring for a child with ADHD: 21 tips" by Jamie Crawford describes person-centred
approaches that parents can use to support a child with ADHD: https://www
.medicalnewstoday.com/articles/321621.php.

CHEO's online resources on learning disabilities include links to books and pamphlets: https://www.cheo.on.ca/en/resources-and-support/learning-disabilities
-and-dyslexia.aspx.

KidsHealth.org, an educational website from The Nemours Foundation, contains
resources and tools divided into sections for parents, kids, and teens. Content
on the site is approved by medical experts. This article provides helpful guidance for parents of children with ADHD: https://kidshealth.org/en/parents
/parenting-kid-adhd.html.

Learning Disabilities Association of America (LDA), an advocacy organization created by parents and professionals, provides in-depth information about learning disabilities and related disorders as well as tools for parents and educators:
https://ldaamerica.org/what-do-parents-of-children-with-learning-disabilities
-adhd-and-related-disorders-deal-with/.

"Parenting Tips for ADHD: Do's and Don'ts" from **Healthline.com**, a reputable website
for information on physical and mental health, describes behavior management
techniques to help parents manage their child's ADHD symptoms: https://
www.healthline.com/health/adhd/parenting-tips.

The American Academy of Pediatrics website features articles and updates on
ADHD in English and Spanish: https://www.healthychildren.org/English
/health-issues/conditions/adhd/Pages/default.aspx.

The Institute of Education Sciences (IES) is an independent organization sponsored
by the United States Department of Education that provides general information on evidenced-based treatments of learning disabilities: https://ies.ed.gov
/ncee/wwc/.

Autism Spectrum Disorder

Austistica is a charitable research organization in the United Kingdom that provides updates on new research: https://www.autistica.org.uk/.

Autism Canada is a national organization that conducts advocacy and supports people with autism and their families. Resources on their website include a service directory called Autism Junction as well as information about therapies and interventions: https://autismcanada.org/.

Autism Science Foundation, an American nonprofit organization, funds research and works to increase public awareness and understanding of autism spectrum disorder: https://autismsciencefoundation.org/what-is-autism/treatment-options/.

Centers for Disease Control and Prevention (CDC) in the United States provides news and updates on ASD research and comprehensive resources on their website, including fact sheets, toolkits, and videos. Some content is available in both Spanish and English: https://www.cdc.gov/ncbddd/autism/index.html.

Simons Foundation Autism Research Initiative (SFARI) publishes a monthly newsletter with news and useful information here: https://www.sfari.org/newsletter/.

Further Reading

Given the importance of parental acceptance and affirmation for LGBTQ2S children and adolescents' mental health, we have included resources specific to this group.

Central Toronto Youth Services' "Families in Transition: A Resource Guide for Families of Transgender Youth, 2nd Edition" provides tools and information to help families foster strong bonds with their trans children and to create safe and supportive homes: https://ctys.org/wp-content/uploads/Families-in-TRANSition.pdf.

GenderCreativeKids is a Montreal-based nonprofit organization run by volunteers. Their resource library provides a wealth of information for parents and youth in a variety of formats: https://gendercreativekids.ca/resources/.

Gender: Your Guide: A Gender-Friendly Primer on What to Know, What to Say, and What to Do in the New Gender Culture by Lee Airton, PhD, is an invaluable resource and an authentic and accessible guide to understanding—and engaging in—today's gender conversation.

LGBT Youth Line, a youth-led organization in Ontario, provides anonymous, nonjudgemental peer support to LGBTQ2S youth through talk, text, and instant messaging: https://www.youthline.ca/.

PFLAG Canada, a national charitable organization founded by parents to help families support LGBTQ2S children, offers resources and support on their website, and through their network of local, volunteer-run chapters across Canada: https://pflag.org/.

PFLAG.org in the United States, in addition to conducting advocacy work, has local chapters across the country to help parents and families: https://pflag.org/.

PREVNet is a network of organizations and researchers working to end bullying in Canada with extensive resources online including videos, tip sheets, and tools to deal with cyber bullying: https://www.prevnet.ca/resources. Their "Bullying Prevention and Intervention in the School Environment: Factsheets and Tools" report is a useful resource for educators and families: https://www.prevnet.ca/sites/prevnet.ca/files/prevnet_facts_and_tools_for_schools.pdf.

Glossary

acceptance and commitment therapy (ACT): A type of psychotherapy that has its roots in cognitive behavior and traditional behavior therapy, and encourages individuals to accept challenging emotions and experiences—rather than avoiding or denying or ruminating on them—and to move beyond them regardless.

activation syndrome: An experience of nervous system hyperarousal, characterized by increased activity, disinhibition, restlessness, irritability, and trouble sleeping, associated with selective serotonin reuptake inhibitors (SSRIs) and selective serotonin and norepinephrine reuptake inhibitors (SNRIs) antidepressants.

adverse childhood experiences (ACES): Refers to a traumatic experience that occurred prior to age eighteen that is recalled as an adult. ACES are associated with negative impacts on physical and mental health in adulthood.

agoraphobia: A fear of leaving the house and avoidance of public spaces and crowds.

anorexia nervosa: A type of eating disorder characterized by significantly low body weight, an intense fear of weight gain or persistent behavior that inhibits weight gain, and disturbance in body image and experience of one's body weight or shape. There are two types—one involving only restriction of food intake, and the other involving episodes of binge-eating and/or purging.

antipsychotics, typical/atypical: Psychiatric medications that target symptoms of psychosis—for example, delusions, hallucinations—presumably by reducing transmission of dopamine between nerve cells, as with the typical or older such medications, and in the case of the atypical or newer such medications, additionally by reducing transmission of serotonin between nerve cells, together with other cellular actions.

anxiety: An experience of intense unease, fear, and often physical discomfort, usually triggered by exposure to some sort of perceived threat in our environment that alerts our body's arousal response.

anxiety disorder: A disorder where sufferers are unable to distinguish between dangers that have real, immediate impact and those that don't; instead, they respond with full arousal to situations that most people would view as safe, which prevents them from attaining important developmental tasks and causes them an extraordinary level of distress.

anxiety disorder, separation: Persistent anxiety that prevents children, and sometimes adolescents, from feeling safe apart from their major attachment figures (usually parents), to an extent that impedes them from developing healthy independent social and educational/vocational lives.

anxiety disorder, social: Persistent anxiety that focuses on an irrational fear of being judged, humiliated, and embarrassed in situations involving other people, leading to avoidance of these situations to an extent that leads to significant impairment socially, educationally, and vocationally.

applied behavior analysis (ABA): A type of behavior therapy that uses behavior analysis and a program of rewards to improve cognition and focus, academic productivity, and to decrease problematic behaviors. Used extensively with children with autism spectrum disorder and those with developmental disorders.

Asperger syndrome: This term has been replaced by the diagnostic term *autism spectrum disorder*, without intellectual impairment, and refers to children and young people who have the features of autism without cognitive or language delays.

attention deficit/hyperactivity disorder (ADHD): A neurodevelopmental disorder with onset prior to the age of seven, characterized by a persistent pattern of inattention and/or hyperactivity and impulsivity that interferes with an individual's development and functioning. There is a form of ADHD said to have its onset in adolescence or adulthood, but this is controversial.

autism spectrum disorder (ASD): A neurodevelopmental disorder characterized by persistent deficits in social communication, and a preference for repetitive patterns of behavior, interests, and activities, which may cause significant social and educational/vocational impairment. Onset is usually before three years of age and may or may not be associated with intellectual impairment.

avoidant/restrictive food intake disorder (ARFID): A type of eating disorder that results in a persistent failure to meet one's nutritional and energy needs to an extent that results in medical, psychological, or social impairment.

behavior regulation: This term refers to our ability to manage our behaviors in a way that we don't give in to impulses to behave in ways that harm our health or other people, and to engage in behaviors that advance our personal and societal goals.

behavioral inhibition: This term refers to a temperament type where children consistently show fear and withdraw when confronted with new situations and people.

behavioral insomnia: This refers to a type of sleep disorder involving challenges initiating and maintaining sleep, resulting in significant negative effects for a child and family, where no medical cause exists.

behavioral interventions: Behavioral interventions arose from learning theory (that most human behavior is the result of interactions between an individual and his or her environment) and use its principles to teach and increase helpful behaviors, and to minimize those that are harmful or, in the case of children, interfere with development.

binge-eating disorder: A type of eating disorder characterized by recurrent episodes of rapidly eating amounts of food when not hungry and that are significantly larger than an amount eaten by most people during a similar period of time, and are associated with a sense of being out of control and marked distress.

bipolar disorder, pediatric: Refers to instances where bipolar disorder emerges in childhood and early adolescence. Very early onset refers to children less than thirteen, and early onset to teens thirteen to eighteen who experience their first episode.

bipolar I disorder: A type of bipolar disorder characterized by both manic and depressive episodes.

bipolar II disorder: A type of bipolar disorder characterized by both hypomanic and depressive episodes.

bipolar spectrum disorders: These disorders comprise bipolar I, bipolar II, and cyclothymia, all of which are long-term mood disorders consisting of episodic mood swings. The differences between the subtypes relate to severity and frequency of symptoms.

body-focused repetitive behaviors (BFRBs): These disorders are related to obsessive-compulsive disorder, and consist of repetitive, so-called grooming behaviors, including biting, pulling, scraping, and picking one's skin, hair, and nails. Examples are excoriation (skin picking disorder) and trichotillomania (hair pulling disorder).

borderline personality disorder (BPD): As with other personality disorders, this disorder is not formally diagnosed is not used in children and adolescents. It refers to a long-standing pattern of erratic and unstable moods, behavior, and self-image, characterized by emotional swings and poor impulse control beginning by early adulthood, often resulting in maladaptive substance use, self-harm, and frequent suicidal thoughts and actions. Borderline personality disorder is thought to result from traumatic experiences, adversity, and/or damaging childhood relationships with adults, although there may also be an inherited component.

bruxism: The involuntary grinding of one's teeth and/or jaw while asleep can affect sleep quality and, in some rare cases, result in dental damage. Insomnia can lead to increased bruxism and vice versa. Dental devices such as mouth guards and relaxation strategies are common treatment interventions.

bulimia nervosa: A type of eating disorder characterized by at least a weekly episode of binge-eating, associated with subsequent so-called purging behaviors to avoid gaining weight, such as self-induced vomiting, misusing medications, fasting, or excessive exercise, in an individual whose self-esteem is unhealthily affected by body shape and weight.

circadian rhythm cycle: Your circadian rhythm cycle is your twenty-four-hour clock or sleep-wake cycle.

circadian rhythm sleep-wake disorder: These are sleep disorders where an individual's sleep is misaligned with a sleep-wake cycle.

cognitive: This term describes our intellectual processes—thinking, reasoning, remembering, learning.

cognitive behavior therapy, child- and family-focused (CFF-CBT): A type of cognitive behavior therapy designed for children and families where the child has bipolar disorder. It combines cognitive behavior therapy with psychoeducation (i.e., education provided to individuals seeking mental health services about relevant psychiatric disorders and their treatments), strategies from interpersonal psychotherapy, and mindfulness, in a family-based treatment model.

cognitive behavior therapy for eating disorders (CBT-E): A type of cognitive behavior therapy that includes specific and concrete recommendations for how patients can approach normalizing their food intake and, where relevant, their weight.

cognitive behavior therapy for insomnia (CBT-i): A type of cognitive behavior therapy designed to treat insomnia. CBT-i focuses on changing sleep habits and schedules, as well as false beliefs about sleep and insomnia that perpetuate the problem.

cognitive behavior therapy/program (CBT): An evidence-based form of psychotherapy that teaches people about the links between their thoughts, feelings, physical sensations, and behaviors, and how to intervene when negative thoughts and feelings contribute to psychological distress and psychiatric disorders.

cognitive remediation therapy (CRT): The focus of this therapy—which is used in a number of different psychiatric disorders—is to improve cognitive function, including attention, memory, social cognition, metacognition (the ability to think about one's thought processes), and executive function.

compulsions: This term refers to behaviors that an individual feels an irresistible urge to perform or feels acute discomfort if unable to do so.

conduct disorder: Refers to a chronic behavioral pattern of ignoring other people's rights and societal rules in adolescents under the age of eighteen. Includes aggression, property destruction, lying, stealing, and violating rules.

continuous airway positive pressure (CPAP) machine: A device that blows a continuous stream of compressed air into the throat, using a mask attached to a tube that connects to a portable machine, and thereby prevents the airway from narrowing. Used in individuals with obstructive sleep apnea to improve their breathing while asleep, and therefore their sleep.

cortisol: A type of hormone that plays roles in the body's stress response, immune response, metabolism, and growth and reproductive processes.

cyclothymic disorder (or cyclothymia): A type of bipolar spectrum disorder lasting at least two years (a year in children and adolescents) with hypomanic and depressive symptoms (but not discrete episodes) for at least half the time and without a symptom-free period of more than two months.

delayed sleep phase disorder (DSPD): A type of circadian rhythm sleep-wake disorder where the person has a pattern of delayed falling asleep and waking that interferes with her desired or prior conventional sleep pattern (in other words, that accommodates daytime work or school).

delusions: Fixed irrational beliefs that may be bizarre (situations that cannot occur in real life) or involve situations that could happen (such as a spouse having an affair or colleagues plotting against you) but where there is absolutely no evidence to support this.

depression, clinical: Also known as a major depressive episode or major depressive disorder, characterized by some or all of the following: sadness; emptiness and hopelessness; irritability; loss of interest in life; sleep and appetite disturbance; disturbances of thinking; agitation; slowed thinking, speech, and movement;

suicidal thoughts; guilty and self-blaming rumination. These symptoms last for most of the day and for more than two weeks and cause problems in many aspects of a person's life.

depressive disorder: (see depression, clinical) Refers to a single episode or recurrent episodes of major depression.

developmental coordination disorders: Refers to lack of ability of both gross motor and fine motor skills expected for one's age and compared with one's peers, to an extent that interferes with the developmental tasks expected at a given age.

diagnosis: Refers to the process of identifying a disease from its signs (found on objective physical examination and investigative tests) and symptoms (experienced by a patient).

dialectical behavior therapy (DBT): A psychotherapy that combines elements of CBT and traditional Eastern meditative practices to help patients learn to manage their emotions and replace self-destructive coping strategies with more adaptive ones.

diaphragmatic breathing: Also called abdominal breathing. Refers to deep breathing using the large, dome-shaped muscle at the base of the lungs, the diaphragm, which slows your breathing rate, makes breathing more efficient. Often recommended as an antidote for fast, shallow breathing associated with anxiety and stress.

dopamine: A neurotransmitter (a chemical that transmits signals between nerve cells in the brain) that has been implicated in psychosis, Parkinson's disease, and our pleasure responses.

dyslexia: A popular term that refers to a learning disorder characterized by problems recognizing and decoding words and poor spelling. The term has been generally replaced by the more general term *learning disorder or disability*.

dysthymia/persistent depressive disorder: This is a type of depressive disorder where a person's mood is depressed for most of the time over a period of two years, or depressed or irritable for one year in children and adolescents, without a symptom-free period lasting more than two months.

eating disorder: Mental illnesses in which individuals experience a level of disturbance in their eating behaviors and associated thoughts and feelings that affect their medical and/or psychological health. People suffering from eating disorders are usually (but not always) overly preoccupied with their eating and weight and shape.

emotional dysregulation: An inability to respond flexibly and constructively to negative emotions.

emotional self-regulation: A person's capacity to manage and respond to emotional experiences in a constructive and adaptive way.

enuresis: Frequent urination in bed or in clothes, after the age of five (or equivalent developmental stage), which causes sleep problems and/or impairment and distress during daytime activities. It can be voluntary or involuntary.

family-based treatment (FBT): A form of family therapy that originated in the Maudsley Institute in London. It is associated with treatment for eating disorders that gives parents primary responsibility to help their child with an eating disorder to restore weight through improved nutrition.

family-focused therapy (FFT): A form of family therapy that brings together education for patients and families about the patient's illness and therapeutic interventions to improve relationships among family members.

generalized anxiety disorder (GAD): A type of anxiety disorder where for most days, for more than six months, a person is unable to control his or her worry and its physical manifestations to an extent that causes significant distress and difficulty functioning socially and at work/school.

growth retardation: Refers to a fetus, infant, or child who fails to develop according to his or her genetically determined potential height and weight.

hallucinations: Disturbances in perception, where someone hears, sees, tastes, feels, or smells something that isn't really there.

hallucinations, hypnagogic: Disturbances in perception, where someone hears, sees, or smells something that isn't really there, that occur when falling asleep.

hallucinations, hypnopompic: Disturbances in perception, where someone hears, sees, or smells something that isn't really there, that occur when waking up.

heritability: A statistic that measures the extent to which variation in a given trait, skill, or physical characteristic can be attributed to genetic factors rather than to environmental influences.

hypersomnolence: Excessive daytime sleepiness, caused most often by poor or inadequate sleep at night, but it can also be the result of some mood disorders and medical conditions.

hypomania: A less severe form of mania characterized by abnormally and persistently elevated or irritable mood and increased energy. Hypomania usually doesn't require hospitalization or entail significant distress or impaired function for the individual experiencing it. Characterizes, together with episodes of major depression, bipolar II disorder.

inpatient (treatment): This refers to treatment delivered in a hospital or residential treatment setting.

interpersonal therapy (IPT): A form of psychotherapy used for depression that focuses on a person's beliefs about and relationships with other people.

intrauterine malnutrition: Refers to the failure of a fetus to receive adequate nutrition, usually because of impaired placental function, leading to poor growth.

lanugo: Fine, unpigmented body hair found in newborns and individuals with anorexia nervosa.

learning disorders: Refers to a pattern of difficulty acquiring and using a skill, sometimes such as reading, writing, numeracy, or nonverbal skills, that is incongruent with a child's age and overall intelligence.

mania: Abnormally and persistently elevated or irritable mood and increased energy that are sufficiently severe to require hospitalization because of risk to self or others or because psychotic symptoms are present. Characterizes, together with episodes of major depression, bipolar I disorder.

medical cannabinoids: These strains of cannabis contain little or none of its psychoactive component, THC, which causes the "high" associated with recreational use, and have more of the component CBD, or cannabidiol, which has little or no effect on an individual's mental state. While there is some evidence suggesting benefit in other medical disorders—chemotherapy-induced nausea in children being treated for cancer, and perhaps in the treatment of epilepsy—there is currently insufficient evidence to suggest benefit for any type of psychiatric disorder.

mental illness (interchangeable with child or adolescent psychiatric disorder): Health conditions involving changes in thoughts, emotions, perceptions, and behavior, associated with distress and/or problems in functioning.

mood disorder: A mental illness that causes an individual to experience sustained and distinct periods of alteration in their emotions, thinking, and bodily functions (sleep, appetite, and energy); these episodes affect sufferers' outlook on themselves, their relationships and work, and the larger world.

mood disorder, substance-induced: Refers to a bipolar spectrum disorder or depressive disorder caused by a prescription or over-the-counter medication, or recreational drug.

mood stabilizers: Medications used in bipolar spectrum disorders and sometimes in hard-to-treat depressive disorders to prevent manic and depressive mood swings. Lithium (Lithium Carbonate ER, Lithobid, Eskalith) is a common and effective mood stabilizer.

motivational enhancement therapy (MET): A short-term therapy originally used for smoking cessation, now used more widely and particularly for substance use disorders, that provides an individual with feedback about her substance use and explores and uses her personal motivation to seek and succeed in treatment.

narcolepsy: A rare sleep disorder characterized by excessive daytime sleepiness. Symptoms can include cataplexy (sudden, involuntary muscle weakness that can cause the person to collapse, usually triggered by strong emotion) and sleep paralysis (a temporary inability to move that usually occurs when falling asleep or waking).

neurodevelopmental disorders: Refers to a group of disorders that affect the very early development of the central nervous system. These include neuropsychiatric disorders such as autism spectrum disorder and ADHD, learning disorders (language, nonverbal, mathematics), impaired motor function, and intellectual disabilities.

neuropsychiatric syndrome: Medical conditions that involve both neurological and psychiatric symptoms. Examples are seizures, ADHD, eating disorders, substance use disorders, and concussion syndromes.

non-rapid eye movement sleep (NREM): NREM sleep is the dreamless part of sleep that consists of four separate stages. During sleep, the body cycles between both NREM and REM (dream part of sleep) but cycles usually begin with NREM.

obsessive-compulsive disorder (OCD): A disorder in which the sufferer experiences intrusive and repetitive thoughts—obsessions—that he is unable to get rid of even though he knows the thought does not make sense and is causing him great distress. Many but not all sufferers try to deal with these thoughts with repetitive ritualized behaviors—compulsions—that soothe them.

obstructive sleep apnea (OSA): Sleep apnea refers to a disorder where individuals stop and start breathing repetitively during sleep. There are a number of possible causes. The obstructive type occurs as a result of a person's throat muscles intermittently relaxing and blocking the airway while they sleep. It is frequently associated with snoring.

off-label use: The use of a medication by a health care provider in an age group, at a dose, in a format, or for a purpose for which it has not received official government approval (in Canada, from Health Canada; and in the United States, the Food and Drug Administration). These agencies review all the available scientific data regarding a medication's benefits and risks in the context of its treatment of specific disorders.

oppositional defiant disorder (ODD): Refers to a child who demonstrates a pattern of angry and irritable mood, argumentative and defiant behavior, and vindictiveness in multiple contexts and over a period of at least six months, to an extent that is outside the usual range for the child's developmental stage, gender, and culture, and causes impaired function for the child in multiple domains.

outpatient (treatment): This refers to treatment where the patient does not need to stay in either a hospital or residential treatment facility overnight. May refer to single appointments occurring regularly or to day treatment or day hospital where the patient spends most of a day at a treatment facility but returns home at night.

panic attack: A sudden episode of intense discomfort and fear, accompanied by significant physical symptoms, in the absence of any real danger. Physical symptoms can include heart palpitations, trouble breathing, trembling, dizziness, and changes in body temperature.

panic disorder: Occurs when a person experiences recurrent panic attacks which cause her to feel persistently anxious for more than a month about the possibility of having further panic attacks, and to change her behavior to avoid having more attacks in a way that causes further harm and disturbance to the person's functioning.

parasomnia: Refers to a number of abnormal behaviors that can occur during sleep, such as sleepwalking, nightmares, sleep eating, sleep paralysis, and sleep terrors. They can occur during any part of the sleep cycle.

phobia: An extreme and debilitating fear of a situation or object that is unrealistic or exaggerated that leads to someone restricting his or her life in harmful ways to avoid the situation or object.

physiological: Refers to how the bodies of living things work. The study of physiology is the branch of biology that explores the normal function of a living organism and its parts.

post-traumatic stress disorder (PTSD): A disorder caused by experiencing trauma that manifests in nightmares, intense memories, and so-called flashbacks, where the sufferer feels as though he is reliving the trauma; a hypersensitive arousal response characterized by irritability, hypervigilance, and sleep problems; avoidance of any potential triggers to memories of the trauma; and negative changes in mood and thinking.

prefrontal cortex: The part of the brain that assesses situations more coolly, plans, makes rational decisions, and controls impulses and emotions. It develops fully by a person's midtwenties. Its development and that of other brain functions may be irreversibly damaged by prolonged drug use during adolescence.

progressive desensitization: Also known as systematic or gradual desensitization, this refers to treating an individual with an anxiety disorder by encouraging her to expose herself at levels of increasing proximity to the things that cause her fear while using acquired coping skills to manage her anxiety. An example would be having someone intensely afraid of dogs first look at a picture of a dog, then a video, then be in a room or garden with a dog, and eventually touch a dog.

psychiatric disorder: May also be referred to as a mental illness. Health conditions involving changes in thoughts, emotions, perceptions, and behavior, associated with distress and/or problems in functioning.

psychiatrist: A medical doctor who has completed additional training in the diagnosis and treatment of psychiatric disorders. Can diagnose and prescribe medications. May work in a hospital, clinic, or private practice setting.

psychologist: A mental health professional who has completed graduate training in psychology, and supervised training. Can diagnose and evaluate mental health concerns, including learning problems, and provide therapy. May work in a private practice, clinic, or hospital setting. Not able to prescribe medication.

psychosis: A mental health condition where an individual's thoughts and perceptions are disrupted to an extent where he or she is unable to recognize what is real and unreal. It may involve hearing, seeing, smelling, and believing things that are not real.

psychotherapy: Talk therapy that addresses a broad range of mental illnesses and emotional disturbances. There are a number of different types of psychotherapy.

psychotic-like experiences (PLEs): Refers to magical thinking (believing that an object, action, or circumstance not logically related to a course of events can influence its outcome), delusional ideas, and hallucinatory experiences that are not associated with a full-blown psychotic episode.

rapid eye movement sleep (REM): REM sleep is the dreaming part of sleep. During sleep, the body cycles between both NREM (the dreamless part of sleep) and REM, but cycles usually begin with NREM before progressing to shorter periods of REM (ten minutes to an hour). REM is characterized by sleep paralysis. Infants and young children have higher amounts of REM sleep than older adolescents and adults.

restless legs syndrome (RLS) and periodic limb movement disorder (PLMD): Disorders characterized by an uncomfortable and persistent need to move one's lower limbs, which become worse late in the day or at night, are exacerbated by rest and lack of activity, and cause sleep disturbance.

risk factor: Any attribute, characteristic, or exposure of an individual that increases the likelihood of developing a disease or injury.

rituals, obsessive-compulsive: These can be repetitive behaviors or thought patterns completed in a specific order or way that an individual with OCD performs in order to try to feel "right" or to push away distressing intrusive thoughts or images. Examples are counting to sixty every time she brushes her hair or saying prayers in a certain order and having to start again if the order is interrupted.

schizophrenia: A long-term mental illness affecting less than 1 percent of individuals in North America. Symptoms include delusions, hallucinations, impaired thoughts and concentration, and lack of motivation.

schizophreniform disorder: Similar to schizophrenia, schizophreniform disorder is a mental illness with symptoms that include delusions, hallucinations, impaired thoughts and concentration, and lack of motivation. However, its duration is between one to six months.

selective serotonin reuptake inhibitors (SSRIs): Medications that increase the amount of serotonin available in the brain by blocking its reabsorption by nerve cells. SSRIs are used primarily to treat depression and anxiety.

sensory defensiveness: Sometimes referred to as tactile defensiveness, this is a term used by occupational therapists to describe a child or adult who may react negatively to touch, textures, sounds, and smells. It is associated with neurodevelopmental disorders such as ASD and, to a lesser extent, to childhood anxiety disorders.

sensory trigger: Refers to a sensation received by the five senses that a child or adult with an extreme sensitivity to certain sensations or with sensory defensiveness experiences as aversive and which causes extreme anxiety.

serotonin: A neurotransmitter, a chemical that transmits signals between nerve cells in the brain and other parts of the body, which has been implicated in depression, anxiety, the digestive system, and the blood clotting pathway.

sleep disorder: Disruptions and/or changes in someone's sleep pattern that negatively affect his or her health, safety, and functioning.

sleep hygiene: Refers to a number of habits and practices that promote improved nighttime sleep quality and daytime alertness.

stimulant (medication): These medications, primarily methylphenidate and dextroamphetamine, have various formats (such as short-acting and long-acting, immediate and delayed release) and increase the availability of the neurotransmitters dopamine and norepinephrine in the brain. They are used to treat ADHD and some other psychiatric disorders such as narcolepsy and sometimes depression in older people. They can also be misused by people without these disorders for their stimulant effect.

substance use disorder: Refers to an individual who cannot control his or her intake of alcohol, medication, or other substance, to an extent that causes medical, psychological, social, legal, and vocational harms. Generally, the person requires more and more of the substance in order to achieve its desired effects.

symptoms, medical: Symptoms refer to effects of a disease or disorder that are experienced by the sufferer. Medical symptoms are experienced as originating in the body but can also be caused by anxiety and stress.

trauma: A direct, witnessed, or learned experience of actual or threatened death, serious injury, or sexual violence. Children may experience trauma in the form of painful medical procedures (for very young children), animal bites, serious car accidents, residential fires, acts of individual or mass violence, natural disasters, and physical, emotional, and sexual abuse.

vocational rehabilitation: A series of services tasked with assisting an individual with an injury or disability with their entrance or return to work.

withdrawal syndrome: A time-limited group of symptoms that occur on stopping or reducing use of a psychoactive substance (including some medications) that has been taken repeatedly, usually for a prolonged period and/or in high doses. Indicates a psychological and/or physiological dependence on the substance.

Notes

Introduction

1. World Health Organization. (2018, September 28). Child and adolescent mental health. Retrieved from https://www.who.int/mental_health/mater nal-child/child_adolescent/en.

Anxiety Disorders

1. Marques, L. (2018, July 22). Do I have anxiety or worry: What's the difference? (blog post). Retrieved from https://www.health.harvard.edu/blog /do-i-have-anxiety-or-worry-whats-the-difference-2018072314303.

2. Pérez-Edgar, K., & Fox, N. A. (2005). Temperament and anxiety disorders. *Child and Adolescent Psychiatric Clinics of North America, 14*(4), 681–706. https://doi.org/10.1016/j.chc.2005.05.008.

3. Beesdo, K., Knappe, S., & Pine, D. S. (2009). Anxiety and anxiety disorders in children and adolescents: Developmental issues and implications for DSM-V. *Psychiatric Clinics of North America, 32*(3), 483–524. https:// doi.org/10.1016/j.psc.2009.06.002.

4. Collishaw, S. (2014). Annual research review: Secular trends in child and adolescent mental health. *Journal of Child Psychology and Psychiatry, 56*(3), 370–393. https://doi.org/10.1111/jcpp.12372.

5. Morgan, A. J., Rapee, R. M., Salim, A., Goharpey, N., Tamir, E., Mclellan, L. F., & Bayer, J. K. (2017). Internet-delivered parenting program for prevention and early intervention of anxiety problems in young children: Randomized controlled trial. *Journal of the American Academy of*

Child & Adolescent Psychiatry, 56(5), 417–425. https://doi.org/10.1016 /j.jaac.2017.02.010.

6. Nestadt, G., Samuels, J., Riddle, M., Bienvenu, O. J., Liang, K., Labuda, M., . . . Hoehn-Saric, R. (2000). A family study of obsessive-compulsive disorder. *Archives of General Psychiatry, 57*(4), 358–363. https://doi.org /10.1001/archpsyc.57.4.358.

7. Bolton, D., Eley, T. C., Oconnor, T. G., Perrin, S., Rabe-Hesketh, S., Rijs-dijk, F., & Smith, P. (2005). Prevalence and genetic and environmental influences on anxiety disorders in 6-year-old twins. *Psychological Medicine, 36*(3), 335–344. https://doi.org/10.1017/s0033291705006537.

8. Scaini, S., Ogliari, A., Eley, T. C., Zavos, H. M., & Battaglia, M. (2012). Genetic and environmental contributions to separation anxiety: A meta-analytic approach to twin data. *Depression and Anxiety, 29*(9), 754–761. https://doi.org/10.1002/da.21941.

9. Svihra, M., & Katzman, M. A. (2004). Behavioural inhibition: A predictor of anxiety. *Paediatrics & Child Health, 9*(8), 547–550. https://doi.org /10.1093/pch/9.8.547.

10. Pérez-Edgar, K., & Fox, N. A. (2005). Temperament and anxiety disorders. *Child and Adolescent Psychiatric Clinics of North America, 14*(4), 681–706. https://doi.org/10.1016/j.chc.2005.05.008.

11. Wehry, A. M., Beesdo-Baum, K., Hennelly, M. M., Connolly, S. D., & Strawn, J. R. (2015). Assessment and treatment of anxiety disorders in children and adolescents. *Current Psychiatry Reports, 17*(7), 52. https://doi .org/10.1007/s11920-015-0591-z.

12. Wang, Z., Whiteside, S. P., Sim, L., Farah, W., Morrow, A. S., Alsawas, M., . . . Murad, M. H. (2017). Comparative effectiveness and safety of cognitive behavioral therapy and pharmacotherapy for childhood anxiety disorders. *JAMA Pediatrics, 171*(11), 1049. https://doi.org/10.1001/jama pediatrics.2017.3036.

13. Walkup, J. T., Albano, A. M., Piacentini, J., Birmaher, B., Compton, S. N., Sherrill, J. T., . . . Kendall, P. C. (2008). Cognitive behavioral therapy, sertraline, or a combination in childhood anxiety. *New England Journal of Medicine, 359*(26), 2753–2766. https://doi.org/10.1056/nejmoa0804633.

14. Velting, O. N., Setzer, N. J., & Albano, A. M. (2004). Update on and advances in assessment and cognitive-behavioral treatment of anxiety disorders in children and adolescents. *Professional Psychology: Research and Practice, 35*(1), 42–54. https://doi.org/10.1037/0735-7028.35.1.42.

15. Lebowitz, E. R., Panza, K. E., Su, J., & Bloch, M. H. (2012). Family accommodation in obsessive–compulsive disorder. *Expert Review of Neurotherapeutics, 12*(2), 229–238. https://doi.org/10.1586/ern.11.200.

16. Kodal, A., Fjermestad, K., Bjelland, I., Gjestad, R., Öst, L., Bjaastad, J. F., . . . Wergeland, G. J. (2018). Long-term effectiveness of cognitive behavioral therapy for youth with anxiety disorders. *Journal of Anxiety Disorders, 53*, 58–67. https://doi.org/10.1016/j.janxdis.2017.11.003.

17. Hancock, K., Swain, J., Hainsworth C., Koo, S., & Dixon, A. (2016). Long-term follow-up in children with anxiety disorders treated with acceptance and commitment therapy or cognitive behavioral therapy: Outcomes and predictors. *Journal of Child and Adolescent Behaviour, 4*(5). https://doi.org/10.4172/2375-4494.1000317.

18. Walkup, J. T., Albano, A. M., Piacentini, J., Birmaher, B., Compton, S. N., Sherrill, J. T., . . . Kendall, P.C. (2008).

19. Caring For Kids (2018). *Using SSRIs to treat depression and anxiety in children and youth* (fact sheet). Retrieved from https://www.caringforkids.cps.ca/handouts/using_ssris_to_treat_depression_and_anxiety_in_children_and_youth.

20. Garland, E. Jane, Kutcher, S., Virani, A., & Elbe, D. (2016). Update on the use of SSRIs and SNRIs with children and adolescents in clinical practice. *Journal of the Canadian Academy of Child and Adolescent Psychiatry = Journal de l'Academie canadienne de psychiatrie de l'enfant et de l'adolescent, 25*(1), 4–10.

Substance Use Disorders

1. Thatcher, D. L., & Clark, D. B. (2008). Adolescents at risk for substance use disorders: Role of psychological dysregulation, endophenotypes, and environmental influences. *Alcohol Research & Health: Journal of the National Institute on Alcohol Abuse and Alcoholism, 31*(2), 168–176.

2. American Psychiatric Association. (2013). *Diagnostic and statistical manual of mental disorders* (5th ed.). Arlington, VA: Author.

3. CAMH. (2017). *Ontario student drug use and health survey: Drug use among Ontario students.* Retrieved from http://www.camhx.ca/Publications/OSDUHS/2017/index.html. Note: Starting in Canada, the Ontario Student Drug Use and Health Survey (OSDUHS) is a population-based study of students in Ontario's public high schools between grades seven and twelve (ages approximately fourteen to eighteen), that began in 1977 in Canada's

largest and most diverse province, and captures responses from thousands of students in more than two hundred elementary and secondary schools. The OSDUHS is conducted every two years and is one of the largest and longest ongoing surveys of youth of its kind in the world. Given its size and longevity, the survey is seen as an exceptionally reliable source of information on health risk behaviors, attitudes, and beliefs of adolescents.

4. Office of Population Affairs, US Department of Health and Human Services. (n.d.). *United States adolescent substance abuse facts.* Retrieved from https://www.hhs.gov/ash/oah/facts-and-stats/national-and-state-data-sheets/adolescents-and-substance-abuse/united-states/index.html#footnote-1.

5. Centers for Disease Control and Prevention. (n.d.). *High school YRBS.* Retrieved from https://nccd.cdc.gov/YouthOnline/App/QuestionsOrLocations.aspx?CategoryId=C03.

6. National Institute on Drug Abuse (2016). Teens and E-cigarettes. Retrieved from https://www.drugabuse.gov/related-topics/trends-statistics/infographics/teens-e-cigarettes.

7. Shi, C.-W., & Bayard, M. A. (2011). Abuse of over-the-counter medications among teenagers and young adults. *American Family Physician, 84*(7), 245–250. Retrieved from https://www.aafp.org/afp/2011/1001/p745.html.

8. Vestal, C. (2018, August 24). Teen Xanax abuse is surging (blog post). Retrieved from https://www.pewtrusts.org/en/research-and-analysis/blogs/stateline/2018/08/24/teen-xanax-abuse-is-surging.

9. McQuaid, R. J. (2017, March 9). *Substance use and suicide among youth: Prevention and intervention strategies* (PowerPoint slides). Retrieved from https://www.mentalhealthcommission.ca/sites/default/files/2017-04/suicide_prevention_webinar_march_2017_eng.pdf.

10. Smit, F., Bolier, L., & Cuijpers, P. (2004). Cannabis use and the risk of later schizophrenia: A review. *Addiction, 99*(4), 425–430. https://doi.org/10.1111/j.1360-0443.2004.00683.x.

11. Gobbi, G., Atkin, T., Zytynski, T., Wang, S., Askari, S., Boruff, J., . . . Mayo, N. (2019). Association of cannabis use in adolescence and risk of depression, anxiety, and suicidality in young adulthood. *JAMA Psychiatry, 76*(4), 426. https://doi.org/10.1001/jamapsychiatry.2018.4500.

12. American Academy of Child & Adolescent Psychiatry (2018, March). *Teens: Alcohol and other drugs no. 3* (fact sheet). Retrieved from https://

www.aacap.org/aacap/families_and_youth/facts_for_families/fff-guide
/Teens-Alcohol-And-Other-Drugs-003.aspx.

13. Loke, A., & Mak, Y. (2013). Family process and peer influences on substance use by adolescents. *International Journal of Environmental Research
and Public Health, 10*(9), 3868–3885. https://doi.org/10.3390/ijerph100
93868.

14. Ramirez, R., Hinman, A., Sterling, S., Weisner, C., & Campbell, C. (2012).
Peer influences on adolescent alcohol and other drug use outcomes. *Journal of Nursing Scholarship, 44*(1), 36–44. https://doi.org/10.1111/j.1547
-5069.2011.01437.x.

15. Hawkins, J. D., Catalano, R. F., & Miller, J. Y. (1992). Risk and protective
factors for alcohol and other drug problems in adolescence and early adulthood: Implications for substance abuse prevention. *Psychological Bulletin,
112*(1), 64–105. https://doi.org/10.1037//0033-2909.112.1.64.

16. Jena, A. B., & Goldman, D. P. (2011). Growing Internet use may help explain the rise in prescription drug abuse in the United States. *Health affairs
(Project Hope), 30*(6), 1192–1199. https://doi.org/10.1377/hlthaff.2011
.0155.

17. Kann, L., Olsen, E. O., McManus, T., Harris, W. A., Shanklin, S. L.,
Flint, K. H., . . . Zaza, S. (2016). Sexual identity, sex of sexual contacts, and
health-related behaviors among students in grades 9–12—United States and
selected sites, 2015. *Morbidity and Mortality Weekly Report (MMWR)*, Surveillance Summaries, *65*(SS-9), 1–202. https://doi.org/10.15585/mmwr
.ss6509a1.

18. Hawkins, J. D., Catalano, R. F., & Miller, J. Y. (1992).

19. Barnes, G. M., Reifman, A. S., Farrell, M. P., & Dintcheff, B. A. (2000).
The effects of parenting on the development of adolescent alcohol misuse:
A six-wave latent growth model. *Journal of Marriage and Family, 62*(1),
175–186. https://doi.org/10.1111/j.1741-3737.2000.00175.

20. National Institute on Drug Abuse. (2014, January 14). *Principles of adolescent substance use disorder treatment: A research-based guide.* Retrieved from
https://www.drugabuse.gov/publications/principles-adolescent-substance
-use-disorder-treatment-research-based-guide.

21. Canadian Centre on Substance Use and Addiction. (2014). *Childhood and
adolescent pathways to substance use disorders.* Retrieved from https://www
.ccsa.ca/sites/default/files/2019-04/CCSA-Child-Adolescent-Substance
-Use-Disorders-Report-2014-en.pdf.

22. Canadian Centre on Substance Use and Addiction. (2014).

23. Shakya, H. B., Christakis, N. A., & Fowler, J. H. (2012). Parental influence on substance use in adolescent social networks. *Archives of Pediatrics & Adolescent Medicine, 166*(12), 1132. https://doi.org/10.1001/archpediatrics.2012.1372.

24. Baumrind, D. (1971). Current patterns of parental authority. *Developmental Psychology, 4*(1, Pt. 2), 1–103. https://doi.org/10.1037/h0030372.

25. Maccoby, E. E., & Martin, J. (1983). Socialization in the context of the family: Parent-child interaction. In P. H. Mussen (Series Ed.) & E. M. Hetherington (Vol. Ed.), *Handbook of child psychology: Vol. 4. Socialization, personality, and social development* (4th ed., pp. 1–101). New York, NY: Wiley.

26. Steinberg, L. (2001). We know some things: Parent-adolescent relationships in retrospect and prospect. *Journal of Research on Adolescence, 11*(1), 1–19. https://doi.org/10.1111/1532-7795.00001.

27. Demuth, S., & Brown, S. L. (2004). Family structure, family processes, and adolescent delinquency: The significance of parental absence versus parental gender. *Journal of Research in Crime and Delinquency, 41*(1), 58–81. https://doi.org/10.1177/0022427803256236.

28. Steinberg, L., Elmen, J. D., & Mounts, N. S. (1989). Authoritative parenting, psychosocial maturity, and academic success among adolescents. *Child Development, 60*(6), 1424. https://doi.org/10.2307/1130932.

29. Gray, M. R., & Steinberg, L. (1999). Unpacking authoritative parenting: Reassessing a multidimensional construct. *Journal of Marriage and the Family, 61*(3), 574. https://doi.org/10.2307/353561.

30. Steinberg, L., Mounts, N. S., Lamborn, S. D., & Dornbusch, S. M. (1991). Authoritative parenting and adolescent adjustment across varied ecological niches. *Journal of Research on Adolescence, 1*(1), 19–36.

31. Bahr, S. J., & Hoffmann, J. P. (2010). Parenting style, religiosity, peers, and adolescent heavy drinking. *Journal of Studies on Alcohol and Drugs, 71*(4), 539–543. https://doi.org/10.15288/jsad.2010.71.539.

32. Driscoll, A. K., Russell, S. T., & Crockett, L. J. (2007). Parenting styles and youth well-being across immigrant generations. *Journal of Family Issues, 29*(2), 185–209. https://doi.org/10.1177/0192513x07307843.

33. Knight, J.R. (2018). The CRAFFT 2.1 Screening Interview. Boston Children's Hospital. Retrieved from http://crafft.org/get-the-crafft/.

NOTICE TO CLINIC STAFF AND MEDICAL RECORDS:

The information on this page is protected by special federal confidentiality rules (42 CFR Part 2), which prohibit disclosure of this information unless authorized by specific written consent. A general authorization for release of medical information is NOT sufficient.

© John R. Knight, MD, Boston Children's Hospital, 2018.

All rights reserved. Reproduced with permission.

For more information, contact crafft@childrens.harvard.edu.

34. Knight, J. R., Sherritt, L., Shrier, L. A., Harris, S. K., & Chang, G. (2002). Validity of the CRAFFT substance abuse screening test among adolescent clinic patients. *Archives of Pediatrics & Adolescent Medicine, 156*(6), 607. https://doi.org/10.1001/archpedi.156.6.607.

35. National Institute on Drug Abuse. (2014, January 14).

36. Tanner-Smith, E. E., Wilson, S. J., & Lipsey, M. W. (2013). The comparative effectiveness of outpatient treatment for adolescent substance abuse: A meta-analysis. *Journal of Substance Abuse Treatment, 44*(2), 145–158. https://doi.org/10.1016/j.jsat.2012.05.006.

37. Nock, N. L., Minnes, S., & Alberts, J. L. (2017). Neurobiology of substance use in adolescents and potential therapeutic effects of exercise for prevention and treatment of substance use disorders. *Birth Defects Research, 109*(20), 1711–1729. https://doi.org/10.1002/bdr2.1182.

38. National Institute on Drug Abuse. (2014, January 14).

39. Naar-King, S. (2011). Motivational interviewing in adolescent treatment. *Canadian Journal of Psychiatry, 56*(11), 651–657. https://doi.org/10.1177/070674371105601103.

40. National Institute on Drug Abuse. (2018, January 17). Principles of drug addiction treatment: A research-based guide (3rd edition). Retrieved from https://www.drugabuse.gov/publications/principles-drug-addiction-treatment-research-based-guide-third-edition.

41. Logan, D. E., & Marlatt, G. A. (2010). Harm reduction therapy: A practice-friendly review of research. *Journal of Clinical Psychology, 66*(2), 201–214. https://doi.org/10.1002/jclp.20669.

42. Jiloha, R. (2017). Prevention, early intervention, and harm reduction of substance use in adolescents. *Indian Journal of Psychiatry, 59*(1), 111. https://doi.org/10.4103/0019-5545.204444

43. Hammond, C. J. (2016). The role of pharmacotherapy in the treat-

ment of adolescent substance use disorders. *Child and Adolescent Psychiatric Clinics of North America*, *25*(4), 685–711. https://doi.org/10.1016/j.chc.2016.05.004.

44. Spithoff, S., & Kahan, M. (2015). Primary care management of alcohol use disorder and at-risk drinking: Part 2: counsel, prescribe, connect. *Canadian Family Physician Medecinde famille canadien*, *61*(6), 515–521.

45. Myers, M. G., & Kelly, J. F. (2006). Cigarette smoking among adolescents with alcohol and other drug use problems. *Alcohol Research & Health: The Journal of the National Institute on Alcohol Abuse and Alcoholism*, *29*(3), 221–227.

46. Harvey, J., & Chadi, N. (2016). Strategies to promote smoking cessation among adolescents. *Paediatrics & Child Health*, *21*(4), 201–204. https://doi.org/10.1093/pch/21.4.201.

47. Auerswald, C. L., Lin, J. S., & Parriott, A. (2016). Six-year mortality in a street-recruited cohort of homeless youth in San Francisco, California. *PeerJ*, *4*, e.1909. https://doi.org/10.7717/peerj.1909.

48. Auerswald, C. L., & Goldblatt, A. (2016). Stigmatizing beliefs regarding street-connected children and youth. *JAMA Pediatrics*, *170*(5), 419. https://doi.org/10.1001/jamapediatrics.2016.0161.

Eating Disorders

1. National Institute of Mental Health. (2016, February). Eating disorders. Retrieved from https://www.nimh.nih.gov/health/topics/eating-disorders/index.shtml.

2. Dieting: Information for teens. (2004). *Paediatrics & Child Health*, *9*(7), 495–496. https://doi.org/10.1093/pch/9.7.495.

3. National Institute of Mental Health. (2017). *Prevalence of eating disorders in adolescents*. Retrieved from https://www.nimh.nih.gov/health/statistics/eating-disorders.shtml#part_155062.

4. Government of Canada (2006). *The human face of mental health and mental illness in Canada, 2006*. Retrieved from http://publications.gc.ca/collections/Collection/HP5-19-2006E.pdf.

5. Sullivan, P. (2002). Course and outcome of anorexia nervosa and bulimia nervosa. In Fairburn, C. G., & Brownell, K. D. (Eds.), *Eating Disorders and Obesity* (pp. 226–232). New York, NY: Guilford.

6. Campbell, K., & Peebles, R. (2014). Eating disorders in children and

adolescents: State of the art review. *Pediatrics, 134*(3), 582–592. https://doi.org/10.1542/peds.2014-0194.

7. Fassino, S. (2017, February 28). Eating disorders: The importance of early intervention (blog post). Retrieved from http://blogs.biomedcentral.com/bmcseriesblog/2017/02/27/eating-disorders-importance-early-intervention.

8. Mohr, H. M., Röder, C., Zimmermann, J., Hummel, D., Negele, A., & Grabhorn, R. (2011). Body image distortions in bulimia nervosa: Investigating body size overestimation and body size satisfaction by fMRI. *NeuroImage, 56*(3), 1822–1831. https://doi.org/10.1016/j.neuroimage.2011.02.069.

9. Carter, J. C., Stewart, D. A., Dunn, V. J., & Fairburn, C. G. (1997). Primary prevention of eating disorders: Might it do more harm than good? *International Journal of Eating Disorders, 22*(2), 167–172. https://doi.org/10.1002/(SICI)1098-108X(199709)22:2167::AID-EAT83.0.CO;2-D.

10. Fairburn, C. G., Doll, H. A., Welch, S. L., Hay, P. J., Davies, B. A., & O'Connor, M. E. (1998). Risk factors for binge eating disorder. *Archives of General Psychiatry, 55*(5), 425–432. https://doi.org/10.1001/archpsyc.55.5.425.

11. Fairburn, C. G., Welch, S. L., Doll, H. A., Davies, B. A., & O'Connor, M. E. (1997). Risk factors for bulimia nervosa. *Archives of General Psychiatry, 54*(6), 509–517. https://doi.org/10.1001/archpsyc.1997.01830180015003.

12. Pike, K. M., Wilfley, D., Hilbert, A., Fairburn, C. G., Dohm, F., & Striegel-Moore, R. H. (2006). Antecedent life events of binge-eating disorder. *Psychiatry Research, 142*(1), 19–29. https://doi.org/10.1016/j.psychres.2005.10.006.

13. Mayhew, A. J., Pigeyre, M., Couturier, J., & Meyre, D. (2017). An evolutionary genetic perspective of eating disorders. *Neuroendocrinology, 106*(3), 292–306. https://doi.org/10.1159/000484525.

14. Campbell, K., & Peebles, R. (2014).

15. Diemer, E. W., Hughto, J. M., Gordon, A. R., Guss, C., Austin, S. B., & Reisner, S. L. (2018). Beyond the binary: Differences in eating disorder prevalence by gender identity in a transgender sample. *Transgender Health, 3*(1), 17–23. https://doi.org/10.1089/trgh.2017.0043.

16. Diemer, E. W., Grant, J. D., Munn-Chernoff, M. A., Patterson, D. A., & Duncan, A. E. (2015). Gender identity, sexual orientation, and eating-

related pathology in a national sample of college students. *Journal of Adolescent Health, 57*(2), 144–149. https://doi.org/10.1016/j.jadohealth .2015.03.003.

17. Hawkins, N., Richards, P. S., Granley, H. M., & Stein, D. M. (2004). The impact of exposure to the thin-ideal media image on women. *Eating Disorders, 12*(1), 35–50. https://doi.org/10.1080/10640260490267751.

18. Witcomb, G. L., Arcelus, J. L., & Chen, J. L. (2013). Can cognitive dissonance methods developed in the West for combatting the "thin ideal" help slow the rapidly increasing prevalence of eating disorders in non-Western cultures? *Shanghai Archives of Psychiatry, 25*(6), 332–340. https://doi.org /10.3969/j.issn.1002-0829.2013.06.002.

19. Diemer, E. W., Grant, J. D., Munn-Chernoff, M. A., Patterson, D. A., & Duncan, A. E. (2015). Note: That transgender men want to appear less curvy and more muscular and transgender women want to appear smaller, thinner, and "more delicate."

20. Campbell, K., & Peebles, R. (2014).

21. UNC Health Talk. (2016, June 2). UNC researchers share "nine truths" for World Eating Disorders Action Day. Retrieved from https://health talk.unchealthcare.org/unc-researchers-share-2018nine-truths2019-for -world-eating-disorders-action-day.

22. Biederman, J., Ball, S. W., Monuteaux, M. C., Surman, C. B., Johnson, J. L., & Zeitlin, S. (2007). Are girls with ADHD at risk for eating disorders? Results from a controlled, five-year prospective study. *Journal of Developmental & Behavioral Pediatrics, 28*(4), 302–307. https://doi.org/10 .1097/dbp.0b013e3180327917.

23. Mikami, A. Y., Hinshaw, S. P., Patterson, K. A., & Lee, J. C. (2008). Eating pathology among adolescent girls with attention-deficit/hyperactivity disorder. *Journal of Abnormal Psychology, 117*(1), 225–235. https://doi.org /10.1037/0021-843x.117.1.225.

24. Cleveland Clinic. (2018, April 24). *How to overcome your child's picky eating habits*. Retrieved from https://health.clevelandclinic.org/how-to-over come-your-childs-picky-eating-habits.

25. Satter, E. (n.d.). *Raise a healthy child who is a joy to feed*. Retrieved from https://www.ellynsatterinstitute.org/how-to-feed/the-division-of-respon sibility-in-feeding/.

26. Sears, W. (n.d.). *Importance of grow foods for children*. Retrieved from

https://www.askdrsears.com/topics/feeding-eating/family-nutrition/grow -food-nutrtip.

27. Rienecke, R. D. (2017). Family-based treatment of eating disorders in adolescents: Current insights. *Adolescent Health, Medicine and Therapeutics, 8*, 69–79. https://doi.org/10.2147/AHMT.S115775.

28. Rienecke, R. D. (2017).

29. Grave, R. D., Sartirana, M., & Calugi, S. (2019). Enhanced cognitive behavioral therapy for adolescents with anorexia nervosa: Outcomes and predictors of change in a real-world setting. *International Journal of Eating Disorders, 52*(9), 1042–1046. https://doi.org/10.1002/eat.23122.

30. Murphy, R., Straebler, S., Cooper, Z., & Fairburn, C. G. (2010). Cognitive behavioral therapy for eating disorders. *Psychiatric Clinics of North America, 33*(3), 611–627. https://doi.org/10.1016/j.psc.2010.04.004.

31. Tchanturia, K., Davies, H., Reeder, C., & Wykes, T. (2010). Cognitive remediation therapy for anorexia nervosa. Retrieved from https://www.national.slam.nhs.uk/wp-content/uploads/2014/04/Cognitive-remediation -therapy-for-Anorexia-Nervosa-Kate-Tchantura.pdf.

32. Robinson, A. L., Dolhanty, J., & Greenberg, L. (2013). Emotion-focused family therapy for eating disorders in children and adolescents. *Clinical Psychology & Psychotherapy, 22*(1), 75–82. https://doi.org/10.1002 /cpp.1861.

Sleep Disorders

1. Institute of Medicine (US) Committee on Sleep Medicine and Research. (2006). Sleep physiology. In Colten, H. R., & Altevogt, B. M. (Eds.), *Sleep disorders and sleep deprivation: An unmet public health problem.* Washington, DC: Author. Retrieved from https://www.ncbi.nlm.nih.gov/books /NBK19956/.

2. Vriend, J., & Corkum, P. (2011). Clinical management of behavioral insomnia of childhood. *Psychology Research and Behavior Management, 4*, 69–79. https://doi.org/10.2147/prbm.s14057.

3. Mindell, J. A., Emslie, G., Blumer, J., Genel, M., Glaze, D., Ivanenko, A., . . . Banas, B. (2006). Pharmacologic management of insomnia in children and adolescents: Consensus statement. *Pediatrics, 117*(6). https://doi.org /10.1542/peds.2005-1693.

4. American Academy of Child & Adolescent Psychiatry (2018, June).

Sleep problems no. 34 (fact sheet). Retrieved from https://www.aacap.org /AACAP/Families_and_Youth/Facts_for_Families/FFF-Guide/Childrens -Sleep-Problems-034.aspx.

5. Leinum, C. J., Dopp, J. M., & Morgan, B. J. (2009). Sleep-disordered breathing and obesity. *Nutrition in Clinical Practice, 24*(6), 675–687. https://doi.org/10.1177/0884533609351532.

6. Cleveland Clinic. (2019, April 22). *Put the phone away! 3 reasons why looking at it before bed is a bad habit.* Retrieved from https://health.cleve landclinic.org/put-the-phone-away-3-reasons-why-looking-at-it-before -bed-is-a-bad-habit/.

7. Adams, S. K., Daly, J. F., & Williford, D. N. (2013). Adolescent sleep and cellular phone use: Recent trends and implications for research. *Health Services Insights, 6*, 99–103. https://doi.org/10.4137/HSI.S11083.

8. National Institute of Neurological Disorders and Stroke. (2019, August 13). *Brain basics: Understanding sleep.* NIH Publication No. 17-3440c. Retrieved from https://www.ninds.nih.gov/Disorders/Patient-Caregiver -Education/Understanding-Sleep.

9. Cortese, S., Faraone, S. V., Konofal, E., & Lecendreux, M. (2009). Sleep in children with attention-deficit/hyperactivity disorder: Meta-analysis of subjective and objective studies. *Journal of the American Academy of Child & Adolescent Psychiatry, 48*(9), 894–908. https://doi.org/10.1097 /chi.0b013e3181ac09c9.

10. Gradisar, M., Jackson, K., Spurrier, N. J., Gibson, J., Whitham, J., Wil-liams, A. S., . . . Kennaway, D. J. (2016). Behavioral interventions for infant sleep problems: A randomized controlled trial. *Pediatrics, 137*(6), pii: e20151486. https://doi.org/10.1542/peds.2015-1486.

11. John Hopkins Medicine. (n.d.). Sleep Study. Retrieved from https://www .hopkinsmedicine.org/health/treatment-tests-and-therapies/sleep-study.

12. Durand, V. M., & Mindell, J. A. (1999). Behavioral intervention for childhood sleep terrors. *Behavior Therapy, 30*(4), 705–715. https://doi.org /10.1016/s0005-7894(99)80034-3.

13. Stanford Health Care. (n.d). Stimulus control. Retrieved from https:// stanfordhealthcare.org/medical-treatments/c/cognitive-behavioral-ther apy-insomnia/procedures/stimulus-control.html.

14. Leinum, C. J., Dopp, J. M., & Morgan, B. J. (2009). Sleep-disordered breathing and obesity. *Nutrition in Clinical Practice, 24*(6), 675–687. https://doi.org/10.1177/0884533609351532.

15. Eick, A. P. T., Blumer, J. L., & Reed, M. D. (2001). Safety of antihistamines in children. *Drug Safety*, *24*(2), 119–147. https://doi.org/10.2165/00002018-200124020-00003.

16. Cummings, C. (2012). Melatonin for the management of sleep disorders in children and adolescents. *Paediatrics and Child Health*, *17*(6), 331–333. https://doi.org/10.1093/pch/17.6.331.

17. Picchietti, D., Allen, R. P., Walters, A. S., Davidson, J. E., Myers, A., & Ferini-Strambi, L. (2007). Restless legs syndrome: Prevalence and impact in children and adolescents—The Peds REST Study. *Pediatrics*, *120*(2), 253–266. https://doi.org/10.1542/peds.2006-2767.

18. Picchietti, M. A., & Picchietti, D. L. (2008). Restless Legs Syndrome and periodic limb movement disorder in children and adolescents. *Seminars in Pediatric Neurology*, *15*(2), 91–99. https://doi.org/10.1016/j.spen.2008.03.005.

Depression, Trauma, and Suicidal Thoughts

1. American Academy of Child & Adolescent Psychiatry (2018, June). *Suicide in children and teens no. 10* (fact sheet). Retrieved from https://www.aacap.org/aacap/families_and_youth/facts_for_families/fff-guide/teen-suicide-010.aspx.

2. Miron, O., Yu, K.-H., Wilf-Miron, R., & Kohane, I. S. (2019). Suicide rates among adolescents and young adults in the United States, 2000–2017. *Journal of the American Medical Association (JAMA)*, *321*(23), 2362–2364. https://doi.org/10.1001/jama.2019.5054.

3. Foley, D. L., Goldston, D. B., Costello, E. J., & Angold, A. (2006). Proximal psychiatric risk factors for suicidality in youth: The Great Smoky Mountains Study. *Archives of General Psychiatry*, *63*(9), 1017–1024. https://doi.org/10.1001/archpsyc.63.9.1017.

4. Gould, M. S., King, R., Greenwald, S., Fisher, P., Schwab-Stone, M., Kramer, R., . . . Shaffer, D. (1998). Psychopathology associated with suicidal ideation and attempts among children and adolescents. *Journal of the American Academy of Child & Adolescent Psychiatry*, *37*(9), 915–923. https://doi.org/10.1097/00004583-199809000-00011.

5. Fergusson, D. M., & Lynskey, M. T. (1995). Suicide attempts and suicidal ideation in a birth cohort of 16-year-old New Zealanders. *Journal of the American Academy of Child & Adolescent Psychiatry*, *34*(10), 1308–1317. https://doi.org/10.1097/00004583-199510000-00016.

6. Kelly, T. M., Cornelius, J. R., & Lynch, K. G. (2002). Psychiatric and substance use disorders as risk factors for attempted suicide among adolescents: A case control study. *Suicide and Life-Threatening Behavior, 32*(3), 301–312. https://doi.org/10.1521/suli.32.3.301.22168.

7. Brent, D. A., Perper, J. A., Moritz, G., Baugher, M., Schweers, J., & Roth, C. (1994). Suicide in affectively ill adolescents: A case-control study. *Journal of Affective Disorders, 31*(3), 193–202. https://doi.org/10.1016/0165-0327(94)90029-9.

8. Brent, D. A., Perper, J. A., Goldstein, C. E., Kolko, D. J., Allan, M. J., Allman, C. J., & Zelenak, J. P. (1988). Risk factors for adolescent suicide. *Archives of General Psychiatry, 45*(6), 581–588. https://doi.org/10.1001/archpsyc.1988.01800300079011.

9. Brent, D. A., Perper, J. A., Moritz, G., Allman, C., Friend, A., Roth, C., . . . Baugher, M. (1993). Psychiatric risk factors for adolescent suicide: A case-control study. *Journal of the American Academy of Child & Adolescent Psychiatry, 32*(3), 521–529. https://doi.org/10.1097/00004583-199305000-00006.

10. National Institute of Mental Health. (2016). *Major depression.* Retrieved from https://www.nimh.nih.gov/health/statistics/major-depression.shtml.

11. Korczak, D. J., Ofner, M., Leblanc, J., Wong, S., Feldman, M., & Parkin, P. C. (2017). Major depressive disorder among preadolescent Canadian children: Rare disorder or rarely detected? *Academic Pediatrics, 17*(2), 191–197. https://doi.org/10.1016/j.acap.2016.10.011.

12. Thapar, A., Collishaw, S., Pine, D. S., & Thapar, A. K. (2012). Depression in adolescence. *Lancet, 379*(9820), 1056–1067. https://doi.org/10.1016/s0140-6736(11)60871-4.

13. Mars, B., Heron, J., Crane, C., Hawton, K., Kidger, J., Lewis, G., . . . Gunnell, D. (2014). Differences in risk factors for self-harm with and without suicidal intent: Findings from the ALSPAC cohort. *Journal of Affective Disorders, 168*(100), 407–414. https://doi.org/10.1016/j.jad.2014.07.009.

14. Chesin, M. S., Galfavy, H., Sonmez, C. C., Wong, A., Oquendo, M. A., Mann, J. J., & Stanley, B. (2017). Nonsuicidal self-injury is predictive of suicide attempts among individuals with mood disorders. *Suicide & Life-Threatening Behavior, 47*(5), 567–579. https://doi.org/10.1111/sltb.12331.

15. Olfson, M., Wall, M., Wang, S., Crystal, S., Bridge, J. A., Liu, S., & Blanco, C. (2018). Suicide after deliberate self-harm in adolescents and

young adults. *Pediatrics, 141*(4), pii: e20173517. https://doi.org/10.1542/peds.2017-3517.

16. National Collaborating Centre for Mental Health (2005). *Depression in children and young people: Identification and management in primary, community and secondary care. (Nice Clinical Guidelines, No. 28).* Leicester (UK): British Psychological Society. Available from: https://www.ncbi.nlm.nih.gov/books/NBK56425/.

17. Meyer, I. H. (2003). Prejudice, social stress, and mental health in lesbian, gay, and bisexual populations: Conceptual issues and research evidence. *Psychological Bulletin, 129*(5), 674–697. https://doi.org/10.1037/0033-2909.129.5.674.

18. Becerra-Culqui, T. A., Liu, Y., Nash, R., Cromwell, L., Flanders, W. D., Getahun, D., . . . Goodman, M. (2018). Mental health of transgender and gender nonconforming youth compared with their peers. *Pediatrics, 141*(5), e20173845. https://doi.org/10.1542/peds.2017-3845.

19. Marshal, M. P., Dietz, L. J., Friedman, M. S., Stall, R., Smith, H. A., Mcginley, J., . . . Brent, D. A. (2011). Suicidality and depression disparities between sexual minority and heterosexual youth: A meta-analytic review. *Journal of Adolescent Health, 49*(2), 115–123. https://doi.org/10.1016/j.jadohealth.2011.02.005.

20. Ryan, C., Huebner, D., Diaz, R. M., & Sanchez, J. (2009). Family rejection as a predictor of negative health outcomes in white and latino lesbian, gay, and bisexual young adults. *Pediatrics, 123*(1), 346–352. https://doi.org/10.1542/peds.2007-3524.

21. Meyer, I. H. (2003).

22. Public Health Agency of Canada. (2016). *Suicide prevention framework.* Retrieved from https://www.canada.ca/en/public-health/services/publications/healthy-living/suicide-prevention-framework.html.

23. Statistics Canada. (2019, June 28). *Suicide among First Nations people, Métis and Inuit (2011–2016): Findings from the 2011 Canadian Census Health and Environment Cohort (CanCHEC).* Retrieved from https://www150.statcan.gc.ca/n1/daily-quotidien/190628/dq190628c-eng.htm.

24. Statistics Canada (2019, June 28).

25. Jiang, C., Mitran, A., Miniño, A., & Ni, H. (2015, September). Racial and gender disparities in suicide among young adults aged 18–24: United States, 2009–2013. Retrieved from https://www.cdc.gov/nchs/data/hestat/suicide/racial_and_gender_2009_2013.pdf.

26. Leavitt, R. A., Ertl, A., Sheats, K., Petrosky, E., Ivey-Stephenson, A., & Fowler, K. A. (2018). Suicides among American Indian/Alaska natives—National Violent Death Reporting System, 18 states, 2003–2014. *Morbidity and Mortality Weekly Report (MMWR)*, *67*(8), 237–242. https://doi.org/10.15585/mmwr.mm6708a1.

27. Centre for Suicide Prevention. (2003). Suicide among Canada's Indigenous peoples. Alert #52. Retrieved from: https://www.suicideinfo.ca/resource/indigenous-suicide-prevention/.

28. Chandler, M. J., & Lalonde, C. E. (2008). Cultural continuity as a protective factor against suicide in First Nations youth. *Horizons—A Special Issue on Aboriginal Youth, Hope or Heartbreak: Aboriginal Youth and Canada's Future*, *10*(1), 68–72.

29. Elias, B., Mignone, J., Hall, M., Hong, S. P., Hart, L., & Sareen, J. (2012). Trauma and suicide behaviour histories among a Canadian Indigenous population: An empirical exploration of the potential role of Canada's residential school system. *Social Science & Medicine*, *74*(10), 1560–1569. https://doi.org/10.1016/j.socscimed.2012.01.026.

30. Kirmayer, L. J., Brass, G. M., Holton, T., Paul, K., Simpson, C., & Tait, C. (2007). *Suicide among Indigenous people in Canada*. Ottawa, ON: Indigenous Healing Foundation. Retrieved from http://www.douglas.qc.ca/uploads/File/2007-AHF-suicide.pdf.

31. Stanford Children's Health. (2019). *Posttraumatic stress disorder (PTSD) in children*. Retrieved from https://www.stanfordchildrens.org/en/topic/default?id=post-traumatic-stress-disorder-in-children-90-P02579.

32. Centers for Disease Control and Prevention. (2019, February 26). *Risk and protective factors*. Retrieved from https://www.cdc.gov/violenceprevention/childabuseandneglect/riskprotectivefactors.html.

33. Bahk, Y., Jang, S., Choi, K., & Lee, S. (2017). The relationship between childhood trauma and suicidal ideation: Role of maltreatment and potential mediators. *Psychiatry Investigation*, *14*(1), 37–43. https://doi.org/10.4306/pi.2017.14.1.37.

34. Souza, L. D., Molina, M. L., Silva, R. A., & Jansen, K. (2016). History of childhood trauma as risk factors to suicide risk in major depression. *Psychiatry Research*, *246*, 612–616. https://doi.org/10.1016/j.psychres.2016.11.002.

35. Negele, A., Kaufhold, J., Kallenbach, L., & Leuzinger-Bohleber, M. (2015). Childhood trauma and its relation to chronic depression in adulthood.

Depression Research and Treatment, 2015 (650804), 1–11. https://doi.org /10.1155/2015/650804.

36. Leverich, G. S., Altshuler, L. L., Frye, M. A., Suppes, T., Keck, P. E., Mcelroy, S. L., . . . Post, R. M. (2003). Factors associated with suicide attempts in 648 patients with bipolar disorder in the Stanley Foundation Bipolar Network. *Journal of Clinical Psychiatry, 64*(5), 506–515. https:// doi.org/10.4088/jcp.v64n0503.

37. Souza, L. D., Molina, M. L., Silva, R. A., & Jansen, K. (2016).

38. Niederkrotenthaler, T., Stack, S., Till, B., Sinyor, M., Pirkis, J., Garcia, D., . . . Tran, U. S. (2019). Association of increased youth suicides in the United States with the release of *13 Reasons Why. JAMA Psychiatry.* https:// doi.org/10.1001/jamapsychiatry.2019.0922.

39. Bridge, J. A., Greenhouse, J. B., Ruch, D., Stevens, J., Ackerman, J., Sheftall, A. H., . . . Campo, J. V. (2019). Association between the release of Netflix's *13 Reasons Why* and suicide rates in the United States: An interrupted times series analysis. *Journal of the American Academy of Child & Adolescent Psychiatry*, pii: S0890-8567(19)30288-6. https://doi .org/10.1016/j.jaac.2019.04.020.

40. Shadrina, M., Bondarenko, E. A., & Slominsky, P. A. (2018). Genetics factors in major depression disease. *Frontiers in Psychiatry, 9.* https://doi.org /10.3389/fpsyt.2018.00334.

41. Lieb, R., Isensee, B., Höfler, M., Pfister, H., & Wittchen, H. (2002). Parental major depression and the risk of depression and other mental disorders in offspring. *Archives of General Psychiatry, 59*(4), 365–374. https:// doi.org/10.1001/archpsyc.59.4.365.

42. Rowland, T. A., & Marwaha, S. (2018). Epidemiology and risk factors for bipolar disorder. *Therapeutic Advances in Psychopharmacology, 8*(9), 251– 269. https://doi.org/10.1177/2045125318769235.

43. Qato, D. M., Ozenberger, K., & Olfson, M. (2018). Prevalence of prescription medications with depression as a potential adverse effect among adults in the United States. *Journal of the American Medical Association* (*JAMA*), *319*(22), 2289–2298. https://doi.org/10.1001/jama.2018.6741.

44. Boylan, K., Vaillancourt, T., Boyle, M., & Szatmari, P. (2007). Comorbidity of internalizing disorders in children with oppositional defiant disorder. *European Child & Adolescent Psychiatry, 16*(8), 484–494. https://doi.org /10.1007/s00787-007-0624-1.

45. Saylor, C. F., Williams, K. D., Nida, S. A., Mckenna, M. E., Twomey,

K. E., & Macias, M. M. (2013). Ostracism in pediatric populations. *Journal of Developmental & Behavioral Pediatrics, 34*(4), 279–287. https://doi.org/10.1097/dbp.0b013e3182874127.

46. Boylan, K., Vaillancourt, T., Boyle, M., & Szatmari, P. (2007).

47. Elmaadawi, A. Z. (2015). Risk for emerging bipolar disorder, variants, and symptoms in children with attention deficit hyperactivity disorder, now grown up. *World Journal of Psychiatry, 5*(4), 412–424. https://doi.org/10.5498/wjp.v5.i4.412.

48. Delbello, M. P. (2018). A risk calculator for bipolar disorder in youth: Improving the odds for personalized prevention and early intervention. *Journal of the American Academy of Child & Adolescent Psychiatry, 57*(10), 725–727. https://doi.org/10.1016/j.jaac.2018.07.871.

49. Pepler, D., & Craig, W. (2014). *Bullying prevention and intervention in the school environment* (fact sheet). Retrieved from https://www.prevnet.ca/sites/prevnet.ca/files/prevnet_facts_and_tools_for_schools.pdf.

50. CAMH Bipolar Clinic Staff. (2013). *Bipolar disorder: An information guide [revised edition].* Retrieved from: https://www.camh.ca/-/media/files/guides-and-publications/bipolar-guide-en.pdf.

51. Mcconnell, E. A., Birkett, M., & Mustanski, B. (2016). Families matter: Social support and mental health trajectories among lesbian, gay, bisexual, and transgender youth. *Journal of Adolescent Health, 59*(6), 674–680. https://doi.org/10.1016/j.jadohealth.2016.07.026.

52. Swanson, S. A., & Colman, I. (2013). Association between exposure to suicide and suicidality outcomes in youth. *Canadian Medical Association Journal, 185*(10), 870–877. https://doi.org/10.1503/cmaj.121377.

53. Centers for Disease Control and Prevention. (2019, February 26).

54. Schonfeld, D. J., Demaria, T., & Disaster Preparedness Advisory Council and Committee on Psychosocial Aspects of Child and Family Health. (2015). Providing psychosocial support to children and families in the aftermath of disasters and crises. *Pediatrics, 136*(4), e1120–e1130. https://doi.org/10.1542/peds.2015-2861.

55. West, A. E., Weinstein, S. M., Peters, A. T., Katz, A. C., Henry, D. B., Cruz, R. A., & Pavuluri, M. N. (2014). Child- and family-focused cognitive-behavioral therapy for pediatric bipolar disorder: A randomized clinical trial. *Journal of the American Academy of Child & Adolescent Psychiatry, 53*(11), 1168–1178. https://doi.org/10.1016/j.jaac.2014.08.013.

56. Dorsey, S., Mclaughlin, K. A., Kerns, S. E., Harrison, J. P., Lambert, H. K.,

Briggs, E. C., . . . Amaya-Jackson, L. (2016). Evidence base update for psychosocial treatments for children and adolescents exposed to traumatic events. *Journal of Clinical Child & Adolescent Psychology, 46*(3), 303–330. https://doi.org/10.1080/15374416.2016.1220309.

57. Markowitz, J. C., & Weissman, M. M. (2004). Interpersonal psychotherapy: principles and applications. *World Psychiatry, 3*(3): 136–139.

58. Goldstein, T. R., Fersch-Podrat, R. K., Rivera, M., Axelson, D. A., Merranko, J., Yu, H., . . . Birmaher, B. (2015). Dialectical behavior therapy for adolescents with bipolar disorder: Results from a pilot randomized trial. *Journal of Child and Adolescent Psychopharmacology, 25*(2), 140–149. https://doi.org/10.1089/cap.2013.0145.

59. Fristad, M. (2006). Psychoeducational treatment for school-aged children with bipolar disorder. *Development and Psychopathology, 18*(4), 1289–1306. https://doi.org/10.1017/S0954579406060627.

60. Fristad, M. A., Gavazzi, S. M., & Mackinaw-Koons, B. (2003). Family psychoeducation: An adjunctive intervention for children with bipolar disorder. *Biological Psychiatry, 53*(11), 1000-1008. https://doi.org/10.1016/s0006-3223(03)00186-0.

61. Young, M. E., & Fristad, M. A. (2007). Evidence-based treatments for bipolar disorder in children and adolescents. *Journal of Contemporary Psychotherapy, 37*(3), 157–164. https://doi.org/10.1007/s10879-007-9050-4.

62. Fristad, M. A., Goldberg-Arnold, J. S., & Gavazzi, S. M. (2002). Multifamily psychoeducation groups (MFPG) for families of children with bipolar disorder. *Bipolar Disorders, 4*(4), 254–262. https://doi.org/10.1034/j.1399-5618.2002.09073.x.

63. Miklowitz, D. J., & Chung, B. (2016). Family-focused therapy for bipolar disorder: Reflections on 30 years of research. *Family Process, 55*(3), 483–499. https://doi.org/10.1111/famp.12237.

64. Curry, J., Silva, S., Rohde, P., Ginsburg, G., Kratochvil, C., Simons, A., . . . March, J. (2011). Recovery and recurrence following treatment for adolescent major depression. *Archives of General Psychiatry, 68*(3), 263–269. https://doi.org/10.1001/archgenpsychiatry.2010.150.

65. Perlis, R. H., Ostacher, M. J., Patel, J. K., Marangell, L. B., Zhang, H., Wisniewski, S. R., . . . Thase, M. E. (2006). Predictors of recurrence in bipolar disorder: Primary outcomes from the Systematic Treatment Enhancement Program for Bipolar Disorder (STEP-BD). *American Journal of Psychiatry, 163*(2), 217–224. https://doi.org/10.1176/appi.ajp.163.2.217.

Psychosis

1. National Institute of Mental Health. (2015, August). *First episode psychosis* (fact sheet). Retrieved from https://www.nimh.nih.gov/health/topics/schizophrenia/raise/fact-sheet-first-episode-psychosis.shtml.

2. CAMH. (n.d.). *Psychosis.* Retrieved from https://www.camh.ca/en/health-info/mental-illness-and-addiction-index/psychosis.

3. Kelleher, I., Connor, D., Clarke, M., Devlin, N., Harley, M., & Cannon, M. (2012). Prevalence of psychotic symptoms in childhood and adolescence: A systematic review and meta-analysis of population-based studies. *Psychological Medicine, 42*(9), 1857–1863. https://doi.org/10.1017/S0033291711002960.

4. Wheeler, A. L., & Voineskos, A. N. (2014). A review of structural neuroimaging in schizophrenia: from connectivity to connectomics. *Frontiers in Human Neuroscience, 8,* 653. https://doi.org/10.3389/fnhum.2014.00653.

5. Yung, A. R., Nelson, B., Baker, K., Buckby, J. A., Baksheev, G., & Cosgrave, E. M. (2009). Psychotic-like experiences in a community sample of adolescents: Implications for the continuum model of psychosis and prediction of schizophrenia. *Australian & New Zealand Journal of Psychiatry, 43*(2), 118–128. https://doi.org/10.1080/00048670802607188.

6. Fonseca-Pedrero, E., Santarén-Rosell, M., Lemos-Giráldez, S., Paino, M., Sierra-Baigrie, S., & Muñiz, J. (2011). Psychotic-like experiences in the adolescent general population. *Actas Españolas de Psiquiatría, 39*(3), 155–162. Retrieved from https://www.ncbi.nlm.nih.gov/pubmed/21560075.

7. Valdesolo, P. (2010, October 19). Why "magical thinking" works for some people. *Scientific American.* Retrieved from https://www.scientificamerican.com/article/superstitions-can-make-you/.

8. Lindley, S. E., Carlson, E., & Sheikh, J. (2000). Psychotic symptoms in posttraumatic stress disorder. *CNS Spectrums, 5*(9), 52–57. https://doi.org/10.1017/s1092852900021659.

9. Oconghaile, A., & Delisi, L. E. (2015). Distinguishing schizophrenia from posttraumatic stress disorder with psychosis. *Current Opinion in Psychiatry, 28*(3), 249–255. https://doi.org/10.1097/yco.0000000000000158.

10. National Institute on Mental Health. (2016, April). *Bipolar disorder.* Retrieved from https://www.nimh.nih.gov/health/topics/bipolar-disorder/index.shtml.

11. Keks, N. A., & Hope, J. (2007). Long-term management of people with

psychotic disorders in the community. *Australian Prescriber, 30*(2), 44–46. https://doi.org/10.18773/austprescr.2007.023.

12. Fusar-Poli, P., Cappucciati, M., Bonoldi, I., Hui, L. M. C., Rutigliano, G., Stahl, D. R., . . . Mcguire, P. K. (2016). Prognosis of brief psychotic episodes. *JAMA Psychiatry, 73*(3), 211–220. https://doi.org/10.1001/jama psychiatry.2015.2313.

13. McGrath, J., Saha, S., Chant, D., & Welham, J. (2008). Schizophrenia: A concise overview of incidence, prevalence, and mortality. *Epidemiologic Reviews, 30*(1), 67–76. https://doi.org/10.1093/epirev/mxn001.

14. Saha, S., Chant, D., Welham, J., & McGrath, J. (2005). A systematic review of the prevalence of schizophrenia. *PLoS Medicine, 2*(5), e141. https://doi.org/10.1371/journal.pmed.0020141.

15. Moreno-Küstner, B., Martín, C., & Pastor, L. (2018). Prevalence of psychotic disorders and its association with methodological issues. A systematic review and meta-analyses. *PLoS One, 13*(4), e0195687. https://doi.org /10.1371/journal.pone.0195687.

16. Dapunt, J., Kluge, U., & Heinz, A. (2017). Risk of psychosis in refugees: A literature review. *Translational Psychiatry, 7*(6), e1149. https://doi.org /10.1038/tp.2017.119.

17. Shevlin, M., Mcelroy, E., Christoffersen, M. N., Elklit, A., Hyland, P., & Murphy, J. (2016). Social, familial and psychological risk factors for psychosis: A birth cohort study using the Danish Registry System. *Psychosis, 8*(2), 95–105. https://doi.org/10.1080/17522439.2015.1113306.

18. Newbury, J., Arseneault, L., Caspi, A., Moffitt, T. E., Odgers, C. L., & Fisher, H. L. (2016). Why are children in urban neighborhoods at increased risk for psychotic symptoms? Findings from a UK longitudinal cohort study. *Schizophrenia Bulletin, 42*(6), 1372–1383. https://doi.org /10.1093/schbul/sbw052.

19. Woolf, A. D., Goldman, R., & Bellinger, D. C. (2007). Update on the clinical management of childhood lead poisoning. *Pediatric Clinics of North America, 54*(2), 271–294. https://doi.org/10.1016/j.pcl.2007.01.008.

20. Algon, S., Yi, J., Calkins, M. E., Kohler, C., & Borgmann-Winter, K. E. (2012). Evaluation and treatment of children and adolescents with psychotic symptoms. *Current Psychiatry Reports, 14*(2), 101–110. https://doi .org/10.1007/s11920-012-0258-y.

21. Buka, I., & Hervouet-Zeiber, C. (2019). Lead toxicity with a new focus:

Addressing low-level lead exposure in Canadian children. *Paediatrics & Child Health*, *24*(4), 293. https://doi.org/10.1093/pch/pxz080.

22. Asarnow, R. F., Nuechterlein, K. H., Fogelson, D., Subotnik, K. L., Payne, D. A., Russell, A. T., . . . Kendler, K. S. (2001). Schizophrenia and schizophrenia-spectrum personality disorders in the first-degree relatives of children with schizophrenia: The UCLA family study. *Archives of General Psychiatry*, *58*(6), 581–588. https://doi.org/10.1001/archpsyc.58.6.581.

23. Cardno, A. G., Marshall, E. J., Coid, B., et al. (1999). Heritability estimates for psychotic disorders: the Maudsley twin psychosis series. *Arch Gen Psychiatry, 56(2)*, 162–168. https://doi.org/10.1001/archpsyc.56.2.162.

24. Selten, J.-P., Lundberg, M., Rai, D., & Magnusson, C. (2015). Risks for nonaffective psychotic disorder and bipolar disorder in young people with autism spectrum disorder. *JAMA Psychiatry*, *72*(5), 483–489. https://doi.org/10.1001/jamapsychiatry.2014.3059.

25. Fish, B., & Kendler, K. S. (2005). Abnormal infant neurodevelopment predicts schizophrenia spectrum disorders. *Journal of Child and Adolescent Psychopharmacology*, *15*(3), 348–361. https://doi.org/10.1089/cap.2005.15.348.

26. Clarke, M. C. (2005). The role of obstetric events in schizophrenia. *Schizophrenia Bulletin*, *32*(1), 3–8. https://doi.org/10.1093/schbul/sbj028.

27. Smit, F., Bolier, L., & Cuijpers, P. (2004). Cannabis use and the risk of later schizophrenia: A review. *Addiction*, *99*(4), 425–430. https://doi.org/10.1111/j.1360-0443.2004.00683.x.

28. Di Forti, M., Sallis, H., Allegri, F., Trotta, A., Ferraro, L., Stilo, S. A., . . . Murray, R. M. (2014). Daily use, especially of high-potency cannabis, drives the earlier onset of psychosis in cannabis users. *Schizophrenia Bulletin*, *40*(6), 1509–1517. https://doi.org/10.1093/schbul/sbt181.

29. National Institute for Mental Health in England. (2003, June). *Early intervention for people with psychosis*. Retrieved from http://www.p3-info.es/PDF/NIMHE.pdf.

30. Stevens, J. R., Prince, J. B., Prager, L. M., & Stern, T. A. (2014). Psychotic disorders in children and adolescents: A primer on contemporary evaluation and management. *The Primary Care Companion for CNS Disorders*. pii: PCC.13f01514. https://doi.org/10.4088/pcc.13f01514.

31. Crossley, N. A., Constante, M., Mcguire, P., & Power, P. (2010). Efficacy of atypical v. typical antipsychotics in the treatment of early psychosis:

Meta-analysis. *British Journal of Psychiatry, 196*(6), 434–439. https://doi
.org/10.1192/bjp.bp.109.066217.

32. Kumar, A., Datta, S. S., Wright, S. D., Furtado, V. A., & Russell, P. S.
(2013). Atypical antipsychotics for psychosis in adolescents. *Cochrane Database of Systematic Reviews*, (10): CD009582. https://doi.org/10.1002
/14651858.cd009582.pub2.

33. Cahalan, S. (2012). *Brain on fire: My month of madness.* New York: Simon
& Schuster.

34. Dalmau, J., Armangué, T., Planagumà, J., Radosevic, M., Mannara, F.,
Leypoldt, F., . . . Graus, F. (2019). An update on anti-NMDA receptor
encephalitis for neurologists and psychiatrists: mechanisms and models.
Lancet Neurology, 18(11), 1045–1057. https://doi.org/10.1016/S1474-44
22(19)30244-3.

35. Morrison, A. K. (2009). Cognitive behavior therapy for people with
schizophrenia. *Psychiatry, 6*(12), 32–39.

36. Ising, H. K., Lokkerbol, J., Rietdijk, J., Dragt, S., Klaassen, R. M. C.,
Kraan, T., . . . Gaag, M. V. D. (2016). Four-year cost-effectiveness of cog-
nitive behavior therapy for preventing first-episode psychosis: The Dutch
Early Detection Intervention Evaluation (EDIE-NL) Trial. *Schizophrenia
Bulletin, 43*(2), 365–374. https://doi.org/10.1093/schbul/sbw084.

37. McGurk, S. R., Twamley, E. W., Sitzer, D. I., Mchugo, G. J., & Mue-
ser, K. T. (2007). A meta-analysis of cognitive remediation in schizophrenia. *American Journal of Psychiatry, 164*(12), 1791–1802. https://doi.org
/10.1176/appi.ajp.2007.07060906.

38. Galletly, C., & Rigby, A. (2013). An overview of cognitive remediation
therapy for people with severe mental illness. *ISRN Rehabilitation, 2013*,
1–6. https://doi.org/10.1155/2013/984932.

39. Bauer, I. E., Gálvez, J. F., Hamilton, J. E., Balanzá-Martínez, V., Zunta-
Soares, G. B., Soares, J. C., & Meyer, T. D. (2016). Lifestyle interventions targeting dietary habits and exercise in bipolar disorder: A systematic
review. *Journal of Psychiatric Research, 74*, 1–7. https://doi.org/10.1016
/j.jpsychires.2015.12.006.

40. Ward, P. B., Firth, J., Rosenbaum, S., Samaras, K., Stubbs, B., & Curtis,
J. (2017). Lifestyle interventions to reduce premature mortality in schizophrenia. *Lancet Psychiatry, 4*(7), e14. https://doi.org/10.1016/s2215-0366
(17)30235-3.

41. Dixon, L. B., & Lehman, A. F. (1995). Family interventions for schizo-phrenia. *Schizophrenia Bulletin, 21*(4), 631–643. https://doi.org/10.1093 /schbul/21.4.631.

42. Claxton, M., Onwumere, J., & Fornells-Ambrojo, M. (2017). Do family interventions improve outcomes in early psychosis? A systematic review and meta-analysis. *Frontiers in Psychology, 8,* 371. https://doi.org/10.3389 /fpsyg.2017.00371.

ADHD

1. Georgiades, K., Duncan, L., Wang, L., Comeau, J., Boyle, M. H., & 2014 Ontario Child Health Study Team (2019). Six-month prevalence of men-tal disorders and service contacts among children and youth in Ontario: Evidence from the 2014 Ontario Child Health Study. *Canadian Journal of Psychiatry, 64*(4), 246–255. https://doi.org/10.1177/0706743719830024

2. Hinshaw, S. P. (2018). Attention deficit hyperactivity disorder (ADHD): Controversy, developmental mechanisms, and multiple levels of analy-sis. *Annual Review of Clinical Psychology, 14*(1), 291–316. https://doi.org /10.1146/annurev-clinpsy-050817-084917.

3. Bélanger, S. A., Andrews, D., Gray, C., & Korczak, D. (2018). ADHD in children and youth: Part 1—Etiology, diagnosis, and comorbidity. *Paediat-rics & Child Health, 23*(7), 447–453. https://doi.org/10.1093/pch/pxy109.

4. Thapar, A. (2018). Discoveries on the genetics of ADHD in the 21st cen-tury: New findings and their implications. *American Journal of Psychiatry, 175*(10), 943–950. https://doi.org/10.1176/appi.ajp.2018.18040383.

5. Pivina, L., Semenova, Y., Doşa, M. D., Dauletyarova, M., & Bjørklund, G. (2019). Iron deficiency, cognitive functions, and neurobehavioral dis-orders in children. *Journal of Molecular Neuroscience, 68*(1), 1–10. https:// doi.org/10.1007/s12031-019-01276-1.

6. Vohr, B. R., Davis, E. P., Wanke, C. A., & Krebs, N. F. (2017). Neuro-development: The impact of nutrition and inflammation during precon-ception and pregnancy in low-resource settings. *Pediatrics, 139*(suppl. 1), S38–S49. https://doi.org/10.1542/peds.2016-2828f.

7. Plas, E. V. D., Erdman, L., Nieman, B. J., Weksberg, R., Butcher, D. T., O'Connor, D. L., . . . Spiegler, B. J. (2017). Characterizing neurocognitive late effects in childhood leukemia survivors using a combination of neuro-psychological and cognitive neuroscience measures. *Child Neuropsychology, 24*(8), 999–1014. https://doi.org/10.1080/09297049.2017.1386170.

8. Schachar, R. J., Park, L. S., & Dennis, M. (2015). Mental health implications of traumatic brain injury (TBI) in children and youth. *Journal of the Canadian Academy of Child and Adolescent Psychiatry 24*(2), 100–108. Retrieved from https://www.ncbi.nlm.nih.gov/pmc/articles/PMC4558980.

9. Hvolby, A. (2015). Associations of sleep disturbance with ADHD: Implications for treatment. *Attention Deficit and Hyperactivity Disorders, 7*(1), 1–18. https://doi.org/10.1007/s12402-014-0151-0.

10. Porter, E., & Krans, B. (2017, October 13). *Parenting Tips for ADHD: Do's and Don'ts*. Retrieved from https://www.healthline.com/health/adhd/parenting-tips.

11. SickKids. (2017, June 16). *ADHD: How to help your child at home*. AboutKidsHealth. Retrieved from https://www.aboutkidshealth.ca/Article?contentid=1997&language=English.

12. Snowling, M. J., & Hulme, C. (2011). Evidence-based interventions for reading and language difficulties: Creating a virtuous circle. *British Journal of Educational Psychology, 81*(1), 1–23. https://doi.org/10.1111/j.2044-8279.2010.02014.x.

13. Harpin, V. A. (2008). Medication options when treating children and adolescents with ADHD: Interpreting the NICE guidance 2006. *Archives of Disease in Childhood—Education and Practice, 93*(2), 58–65. https://doi.org/10.1136/adc.2006.106864.

14. Chang, Z., Lichtenstein, P., Halldner, L., D'Onofrio, B., Serlachius, E., Fazel, S., . . . Larsson, H. (2014). Stimulant ADHD medication and risk for substance abuse. *Journal of Child Psychology and Psychiatry, and Allied Disciplines, 55*(8), 878–885. https://doi.org/10.1111/jcpp.12164.

15. Wilens, T. E., Adler, L. A., Adams, J., Sgambati, S., Rotrosen, J., Sawtelle, R., . . . & Fusillo, S. (2008). Misuse and diversion of stimulants prescribed for ADHD: A systematic review of the literature. *Journal of the American Academy of Child and Adolescent Psychiatry, 47*(1), 21–31. https://doi.org/10.1097/chi.0b013e31815a56f1.

Autism Spectrum Disorder

1. Autism Canada. (2017). *Diagnostic criteria—DSM-5/autism spectrum disorder 299.00 (F84.0)*. Retrieved from https://autismcanada.org/about-autism/diagnosis/diagnostic-criteria-dsm-5/.

2. Drmic, I. E., Szatmari, P., & Volkmar, F. (2018). Life course health development in autism spectrum disorders. In Halfon, N., Forrest, C.,

Lerner, R., & Faustman, E. (Eds.), *Handbook of life course health development*. Cham, Switzerland: Springer.

3. Zwaigenbaum, L., & Penner, M. (2018). Autism spectrum disorder: Advances in diagnosis and evaluation. *BMJ, 361*, k1674. https://doi.org /10.1136/bmj.k1674.

4. Reichow, B., Hume, K., Barton, E. E., & Boyd, B. A. (2018). Early intensive behavioral intervention (EIBI) for young children with autism spectrum disorders (ASD). *Cochrane Database of Systematic Reviews, 5*(5), CD009260. https://doi.org/10.1002/14651858.CD009260.pub3.

5. Devlin, B., & Scherer, S. W. (2012). Genetic architecture in autism spectrum disorder. *Current Opinion in Genetics & Development, 22*(3), 229–237. https://doi.org/10.1016/j.gde.2012.03.002.

6. Hviid, A., Hansen, J. V., Frisch, M., & Melbye, M. (2019). Measles, mumps, rubella vaccination and autism: A nationwide cohort study. Annals of Internal Medicine, *170*(8), 513–520. https://doi.org/10.7326 /M18-2101.

7. Bölte, S., Girdler, S., & Marschik, P. B. (2019). The contribution of environmental exposure to the etiology of autism spectrum disorder. *Cellular and Molecular Life Sciences* (*CMLS*), *76*(7), 1275–1297. https://doi.org /10.1007/s00018-018-2988-4.

8. Drmic, I. E., Szatmari, P., & Volkmar, F. (2018).

9. Leaf, J. B., Leaf, R., Mceachin, J., Cihon, J. H., & Ferguson, J. L. (2017). Advantages and challenges of a home- and clinic-based model of behavioral intervention for individuals diagnosed with autism spectrum disorder. *Journal of Autism and Developmental Disorders, 48*(6), 2258–2266. https://doi.org/10.1007/s10803-017-3443-3.

10. White, S. W., Elias, R., Capriola-Hall, N. N., Smith, I. C., Conner, C. M., Asselin, S. B., . . . Mazefsky, C. A. (2017). Development of a college transition and support program for students with autism spectrum disorder. *Journal of Autism and Developmental Disorders, 47*(10), 3072–3078. https://doi.org/10.1007/s10803-017-3236-8.

11. Mcconachie, H., Livingstone, N., Morris, C., Beresford, B., Couteur, A. L., Gringras, P., . . . Parr, J. R. (2017). Parents suggest which indicators of progress and outcomes should be measured in young children with autism spectrum disorder. *Journal of Autism and Developmental Disorders, 48*(4), 1041–1051. https://doi.org/10.1007/s10803-017-3282-2.

12. Russell, G., Kapp, S. K., Elliott, D., Elphick, C., Gwernan-Jones, R., &

Owens, C. (2019). Mapping the autistic advantage from the accounts of adults diagnosed with autism: A qualitative study. *Autism in Adulthood: Challenges and Management, 1*(2), 124–133. https://doi.org/10.1089/aut.2018.0035.

13. Gates, J. A., Kang, E., & Lerner, M. D. (2017). Efficacy of group social skills interventions for youth with autism spectrum disorder: A systematic review and meta-analysis. *Clinical Psychology Review, 52*, 164–181. https://doi.org/10.1016/j.cpr.2017.01.006.

14. White, S. W., Simmons, G. L., Gotham, K. O., Conner, C. M., Smith, I. C., Beck, K. B., & Mazefsky, C. A. (2018). Psychosocial treatments targeting anxiety and depression in adolescents and adults on the autism spectrum: Review of the latest research and recommended future directions. *Current Psychiatry Reports, 20*(10), 82. https://doi.org/10.1007/s11920-018-0949-0.

15. Sturman, N., Deckx, L., & van Driel, M. L. (2017). Methylphenidate for children and adolescents with autism spectrum disorder. *Cochrane Database of Systematic Reviews, 11*(11), CD011144. https://doi.org/10.1002/14651858.CD011144.pub2.

16. Fung, L. K., Mahajan, R., Nozzolillo, A., Bernal, P., Krasner, A., Jo, B., . . . Hardan, A. Y. (2016). Pharmacologic treatment of severe irritability and problem behaviors in autism: A systematic review and meta-analysis. *Pediatrics, 137*(Suppl. 2), S124–S135. https://doi.org/10.1542/peds.2015-2851k.

About the Authors

Pier Bryden, MD, is a psychiatrist and award-winning clinical teacher at The Hospital for Sick Children and an associate professor at the University of Toronto Faculty of Medicine. A graduate of the University of Toronto, Oxford University, and McMaster University, she has published academically and teaches on the ethical and legal aspects of the treatment of children and adolescents with psychiatric disorders. With Dr. David Goldbloom, she is the coauthor of the national bestseller *How Can I Help?: A Week in My Life as a Psychiatrist.* She has two sons.

Peter Szatmari, MD, is the chief of the Child and Youth Mental Health Collaborative between the Centre for Addiction and Mental Health, The Hospital for Sick Children, and the University of Toronto. The head of one of the largest divisions of child and adolescent psychiatry in the world, he also holds the Patsy and Jamie Anderson Chair in Child and Youth Mental Health. He has won awards from several international organizations for his research and is the author of *A Mind Apart: Understanding Children with Autism and Asperger Syndrome.* He has three daughters.